Clinicians' Guide to Li i l
and Coronary Hear

14

Clinicians' Guide to Lipids and Coronary Heart Disease

D.J. Betteridge
Department of Medicine, University College
London,
The Middlesex Hospital, London UK

and

J.M. Morrell
Fitznells Manor Surgery, Ewell, Surrey UK

A member of the Hodder Headline Group
LONDON • SYDNEY • AUCKLAND
Copublished in the USA by
Oxford University Press, Inc., New York

First published in Great Britain in 1998
Reprinted 1999 by Arnold,
a member of the Hodder Headline Group,
338 Euston Road, London NW1 3BH

http://www.arnoldpublishers.com

Co-published in the USA by
Oxford University Press Inc.,
198 Madison Avenue, New York, NY10016
Oxford is a registered trademark of Oxford University Press

British Library Cataloguing in Publication Data
A catalogue record for this book is available from the British Library

Library of Congress Cataloging-in-Publication Data
A catalog record for this book is available from the Library of Congress

ISBN 0 412 75720 6

2 3 4 5 6 7 8 9 10

Typeset in 11/13pt Adobe Garamond by Photoprint, Torquay, Devon
Printed and bound in Great Britain at the Alden Press, Oxford

Contents

Colour plates appear between pages 108 and 109

Preface

This book devoted to lipids and heart disease is extremely timely given the burst of new information which has emerged in the last few years. In a relatively short time the cholesterol/coronary heart disease story has moved from the 'evangelical' and 'the unproven myths of the cholesterol brigade' to evidence-based medicine. It is difficult to think of another area of medicine so rich in understanding of physiology and pathophysiology at a cellular and genetic level with highly effective therapeutic compounds and clinical end point trials performed to the very best standards of clinical trial science. Despite these formidable advances much still needs to be done to educate students and physicians in lipid and lipoprotein metabolism, the relationship to vascular damage, the highly effective treatments which are available and the evidence for their use.

There is often a lag time before proven remedies filter down from research studies to clinical care. Sadly, because of the previous intense controversy about the relative benefits and safety of cholesterol lowering, progress is slow in changing physicians' attitudes and ensuring that patients receive optimal care. Recent surveys still point to gross undertreatment with lipid-lowering drugs which have been shown to improve overall survival. As with all areas of medicine, economic considerations have come to the fore and in the lipid area it appears to the authors that there may be obfuscation of the benefits of cholesterol lowering for financial reasons.

The book is divided into four main parts – Background (information on lipid and lipoprotein metabolism epidemiology and lipid lowering trials); Screening and Assessment; Interventions and Practical Considerations. From our different backgrounds we have brought complementary experience which, hopefully, will enable the interested reader to get a grasp of the subject and, perhaps for a few, sow the seeds for a developing interest.

We have been encouraged in the preparation of this book by our friends and colleagues and have received considerable support from the publishers, particularly Dr Peter Altman. We gratefully acknowledge his help and advice. The book will succeed if its readers are stimulated to take an interest in what is no doubt an important area of medicine, but principally if, as a result, patients receive appropriate therapy based on strong pathophysiological and clinical trial foundation.

D.J. Betteridge
J.M. Morrell

Acknowledgements

To my wife, Chris, and children, Tom and Sally, with much love and thanks for their continuing forbearance; and to my patients, who continue to inspire and challenge me to greater efforts. I gratefully acknowledge my ever-patient personal assistant Jean De Luca for her skill and expertise in the manuscript preparation.

John Betteridge

I would like to acknowledge gratefully the help, support and tolerance of my family, Anne, James and Mark, my secretary, Mrs Olive Rafferty and my colleague and friend Dr Ralph Burton.

Jonathan Morrell

List of abbreviations

ATP	Adult Treatment Panel
BMI	body mass index
BP	blood pressure
BRHS	British Regional Heart Survey
CABG	coronary artery bypass graft
CARE	Cholesterol and Recurrent Events trial
CCF	congestive cardiac failure
CHD	coronary heart disease
CPR	cardiopulmonary resuscitation
CVA	cerebrovascular accident
CVD	cerebrovascular disease
DBP	diastolic blood pressure
EAS	European Atherosclerosis Society
ECG	electrocardiograph
ESC	European Society of Cardiology
ESH	European Society of Hypertension
EWPHE	European Working Party on Hypertension in the Elderly
FCH	familial combined hypercholesterolaemia
FH	familial hypercholesterolaemia
HDL	high density lipoprotein
HHS	Helsinki Heart Study
HRT	hormone replacement therapy
IDDM	insulin-dependent diabetes mellitus
IDL	intermediate density lipoprotein
LDL	low density lipoprotein
LRC	Lipid Research Clinics trial
LVH	left ventricular hypertrophy
MI	myocardial infarction
MONICA	Monitoring Cardiovascular Disease
MRC	Medical Research Council
MRFIT	Multiple Risk Factor Intervention Trial
MUFA	monounsaturated fatty acids
NCEP	National Cholesterol Education Project
NIDDM	non-insulin-dependent diabetes mellitus
OPCS	Office of Population Censuses and Surveys
PROCAM	Prospective Cardiovascular Münster study

PTCA	percutaneous transluminal coronary angioplasty
PUFA	polyunsaturated fatty acids
PVD	peripheral vascular disease
RDB	regression dilution bias
4S	Scandinavian Simvastatin Survival Study
SAFA	saturated fatty acids
SBP	systolic blood pressure
SD	standard deviation
SDE	surrogate dilution effect
SHEP	Systolic Hypertension in the Elderly Program
SMR	standard mortality ratio
TC	total cholesterol
TG	triglyceride
TIA	transient ischaemic attack
TSH	thyroid stimulating hormone
VLDL	very low density lipoprotein
WHR	waist hip ratio
WHO	World Health Organization
WOSCOPS	West of Scotland Coronary Prevention Study

Part One
Background

Lipid and lipoprotein metabolism – the basics

1

It is the authors' experience that colleagues not in the field often have difficulties getting to grips with lipid and lipoprotein metabolism. This area of biochemistry and physiology has perhaps not been well covered at medical school and has been the subject of sometimes confusing and changing nomenclature. This is a pity, as many fundamental and exciting developments have taken place in the last two decades.

Recent advances have provided considerable insight into the control of lipoprotein metabolism, a rational approach to the development of therapeutic agents and an understanding of some of the dyslipidaemias at the molecular level. The latter development has made possible the first attempts at gene therapy in homozygous familial hypercholesterolaemia.

It is not proposed to provide here a detailed description of lipid and lipoprotein metabolism and the enthusiastic reader is directed to several recent and comprehensive reviews in the further reading section. Rather, the basics of lipoprotein metabolism will be described to enable an understanding of the primary and secondary dyslipidaemias, the action of lifestyle and drugs in modulating plasma lipid levels and the role of lipoproteins in atherosclerosis and arterial function.

Lipids and lipoproteins

The two major lipids in plasma – cholesterol and triglyceride – have essential functions in the overall structure and fuel economy of the body.

Cholesterol

In its free, unesterified form (Figure 1.1) cholesterol is a major component (together with phospholipid) of cell membranes. Its presence helps to

Figure 1.1
Structure of free and
esterified cholesterol.

Cholesterol

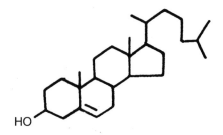

Cholesterol
esters

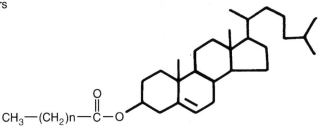

stabilize membrane fluidity and therefore the barrier between cell and
environment. Cholesterol is also important as a precursor of steroid
hormones and of bile acids. Cholesterol present in the plasma and extracellular fluid is largely in the esterified form (Figure 1.1).

Triglycerides
Triglycerides are produced by the esterification of glycerol with three fatty
acid molecules (Figure 1.2). They are the body's major energy store,
particularly in adipose tissue. Fatty acids are released through the action of
hormone-sensitive lipase, an enzyme that becomes active during fasting
when insulin levels are low. They can be utilized directly as fuel by muscle
or, following partial oxidation to ketone bodies in the liver, by other tissues,
including brain.

Figure 1.2
Structure of triglyceride (tri
acyl glycerol) with, for
illustration, (a) a saturated
fatty acid, (b) a mono-
unsaturated fatty acid and
(c) a polyunsaturated fatty
acid.

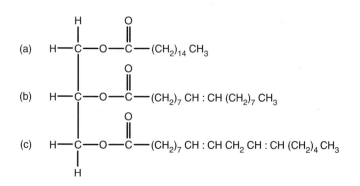

Triglyceride and cholesterol ester are insoluble in the aqueous environment of the plasma and are solubilized by their incorporation into lipoproteins.

LIPOPROTEIN STRUCTURE

There are several different lipoprotein species found in plasma but their basic structures are similar (Figure 1.3). The insoluble lipid (cholesterol ester and triglyceride) forms a central core in the form of a lipid droplet. This is surrounded by an outer monolayer of molecules such as free cholesterol, phospholipids and proteins termed apoproteins which give the complexes their name. These molecules are able to sit at the water/fat interface because they are partly water-soluble and partly lipid-soluble.

Apoproteins

Apoproteins not only stabilize lipoprotein structure but also have other important regulatory functions in lipoprotein metabolism. Apoproteins B_{100} and E are necessary for the binding of lipoproteins to cellular receptors,

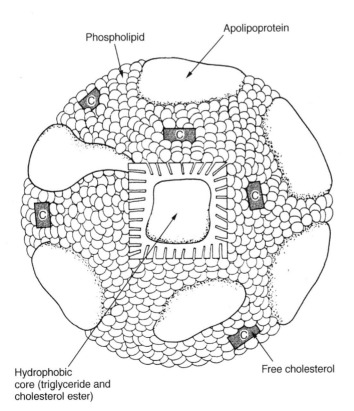

Figure 1.3
Structure of lipoprotein.

Figure 1.4
Plasma lipoproteins.

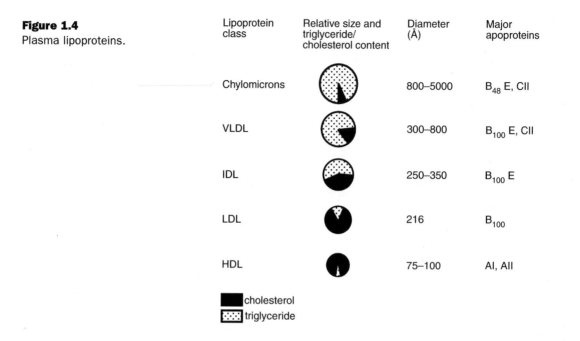

Lipoprotein class	Relative size and triglyceride/ cholesterol content	Diameter (Å)	Major apoproteins
Chylomicrons		800–5000	B_{48} E, CII
VLDL		300–800	B_{100} E, CII
IDL		250–350	B_{100} E
LDL		216	B_{100}
HDL		75–100	AI, AII

■ cholesterol
▦ triglyceride

whereas apoproteins A-I and C-II are activators of enzymes important in lipoprotein metabolism.

LIPOPROTEIN CLASSIFICATION

Lipoproteins are classified predominantly according to their separation in the ultracentrifuge. This separation depends on the hydrated density of the different lipoproteins (Figure 1.4).

Lipoprotein metabolism

Lipoproteins serve to transport absorbed dietary fat and endogenously synthesized cholesterol and triglyceride. The pathways of lipoprotein metabolism are complex and there is much interaction between individual lipoprotein species. Nevertheless, it is possible to provide a relatively simple overview covering three main areas: the exogenous and endogenous pathways and reverse cholesterol transport. In these various pathways the liver has a pivotal role.

EXOGENOUS PATHWAY

In the typical Western diet approximately 80–140 g triglyceride and 0.5–1.5 g cholesterol are eaten daily. Following digestion, absorption and re-esterification, triglyceride and cholesterol are packaged in the jejunal enterocyte with apoprotein B_{48} to form chylomicrons. These are the largest of the lipoprotein species.

Chylomicrons

Chylomicrons enter the circulation via intestinal lymphatics and finally the thoracic duct. Here they acquire additional apoproteins, principally the C group and apoprotein E, which transfer from high density lipoprotein (HDL). They are rapidly metabolized in two discrete phases (Figure 1.5). The large triglyceride component is hydrolysed to fatty acids and glycerol by the lipoprotein lipase enzyme, which is bound to endothelium in capillary beds of muscle and adipose tissue. Apoprotein C-II is an important activator of the enzyme.

The hydrolysis of chylomicron triglyceride by lipoprotein lipase enables the targeted delivery of fatty acids either as fuel in muscle or for re-esterification to triglyceride and storage in adipose tissue. As chylomicron triglyceride is progressively removed some of the surface components of the particle (principally apoproteins and phospholipid) become redundant and transfer to HDL (Figure 1.5).

Chylomicron remnant

The partially hydrolysed chylomicron or remnant is removed by the liver through a high affinity, saturable process which is dependent on apoprotein E in the particle. The most likely hepatic receptor is low density lipoprotein

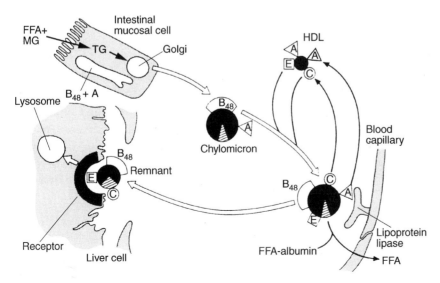

Figure 1.5
Exogenous lipoprotein pathway. FFA = free fatty acid; MG = mono-glyceride; TG = tri-glyceride. Source: Havel, R.J. (1982) *Medical Clinics of North America*, **66**, 319.

(LDL) receptor-related protein (LRP). Proteoglycan and released lipoprotein lipase enzyme also appear to be important in the rapid hepatic uptake of remnants.

In relation to overall cholesterol homeostasis it is important to recognize that the cholesterol component of chylomicrons remains with the particle so that dietary cholesterol is delivered to the liver almost quantitatively.

ENDOGENOUS PATHWAY

Very low density lipoproteins

Triglyceride and cholesterol synthesized in the liver are secreted in very low density lipoprotein (VLDL) particles which serve to transport the lipids to the periphery. VLDL forms a spectrum of particles that differ in size and metabolic fate.

Regulation of hepatic VLDL production is poorly understood. However, it appears that the major VLDL apoprotein, apoprotein B_{100}, is made continuously by liver cells (Figure 1.6). It is degraded in the absence of lipid, which is necessary for lipoprotein assembly to begin. A newly discovered protein called microsomal transfer protein may be important in this process.

Figure 1.6
Endogenous lipoprotein pathway. FFA = free fatty acid; TG = triglyceride. Source: Havel, R.J. (1982) *Medical Clinics of North America*, **66**, 319.

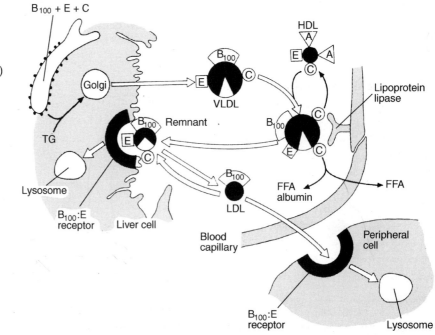

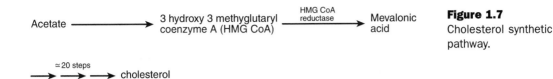

Figure 1.7
Cholesterol synthetic pathway.

The nature of the lipid(s) essential for VLDL assembly remains controversial but cholesterol ester appears to be critical, together with intra-hepatic triglyceride lipolysis to fatty acids and their subsequent re-esterification just prior to the incorporation of triglyceride into the particle.

Hepatic cholesterol synthesis

This is a highly complex process beginning with acetyl CoA formed from fatty acid oxidation or from carbohydrate breakdown. The rate-determining reaction, which is the conversion of hydroxy methyl glutaryl (HMG) CoA to mevalonate, is catalysed by the enzyme HMG-CoA reductase (Figure 1.7). It is the activity of this enzyme that largely determines the rate of cholesterol synthesis.

Hepatic triglyceride synthesis

Fatty acid flux to the liver from adipose tissue appears to be an important determinant of hepatic triglyceride synthesis and VLDL secretion. Hepatic lipogenesis from carbohydrate substrates is also important. In addition, chylomicron remnant uptake makes a significant contribution to the hepatic lipid pool, providing an important interaction between the exogenous and endogenous pathways.

Intermediate density lipoproteins

As with chylomicrons, the triglyceride component of VLDL is hydrolysed by lipoprotein lipase. Resulting VLDL remnants, which like chylomicron remnants share intermediate density (IDL) on ultracentrifugation, are either removed directly by the liver or further metabolized to LDL through the action of hepatic lipase.

LDL

LDL is the major cholesterol-rich lipoprotein carrying approximately 70% of plasma cholesterol. It serves to transport cholesterol to peripheral cells. Much is now understood about how LDL interacts with the cell membrane and its subsequent internalization and regulation of cellular cholesterol homeostasis (Figure 1.8).

The Nobel laureates Brown and Goldstein identified the LDL receptor that recognizes apoprotein B_{100} of LDL particles (Brown and Goldstein,

Figure 1.8
LDL receptor pathway. Increasing cellular cholesterol derived from internalization of LDL decreases HMG CoA reductase activity, activates ACAT and decreases LDL receptor activity. The LDL receptor is formed in the endoplasmic reticulum and travels to the coated pit region of the cell membrane. Source: Brown and Goldstein (1985).

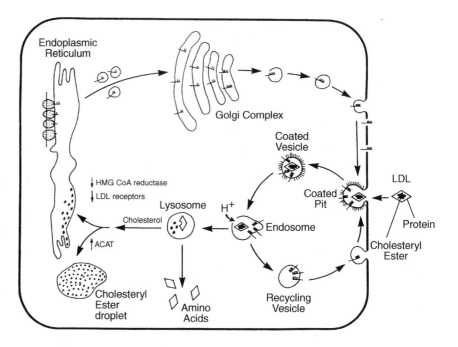

1986). The receptors are large glycoproteins situated on the surface of cells in specialized areas termed coated pits. Coated pits are organelles necessary for the internalization of macromolecules.

The LDL receptor gene has been cloned and localized to the short arm of chromosome 19. The structure (Figure 1.9) and function of the receptor are well understood. The region responsible for binding LDL apoprotein B_{100} is a negatively charged region at the amino terminal end of the molecule which consists of seven repeating units of a 40 amino acid sequence rich in cysteine residues. At the carboxyl-terminal end is a 50 amino acid domain which is responsible for localization of the receptor in the coated pit regions of cell membranes.

The clinical relevance of this structural detail of the receptor will be appreciated when the inborn error of cholesterol metabolism called familial hypercholesterolaemia is discussed. In this condition there are defects in the gene coding for the receptor.

LDL receptor pathway

Following binding, the receptor/LDL complex is internalized by absorptive endocytosis. The endocytotic vesicle fuses with cellular lysosomes where LDL cholesterol ester is hydrolysed to free cholesterol and protein to amino acids. The LDL receptor recycles to the cell surface.

The increasing cellular free cholesterol generated by this process regulates the activities of two enzymes that are of crucial importance in cholesterol homeostasis (Figure 1.8). HMG-CoA reductase (the major rate-determining enzyme in the cholesterol synthetic pathway) is inhibited, reducing cholesterol synthesis. Acyl CoA:cholesterol acyl transferase (ACAT) is activated, thus facilitating the re-esterification of cholesterol to cholesterol ester. In addition the expression of LDL receptors is reduced as cellular cholesterol increases.

Thus the LDL receptor pathway is a closely integrated system by which cells acquire cholesterol and cellular cholesterol homeostasis is maintained. The therapeutic potential of interrupting this pathway will become apparent when the statin drugs which are inhibitors of HMG-CoA reductase are discussed.

It is the activity of LDL receptors in the liver that largely controls plasma LDL levels. Approximately 70% of LDL is removed by this pathway. The importance of the receptor pathway is clear from consideration of the disease familial hypercholesterolaemia (FH) (p.104). LDL receptor activity is substantially reduced in patients heterozygous for FH and virtually absent in homozygotes. As a result the plasma half-life of LDL is extended from

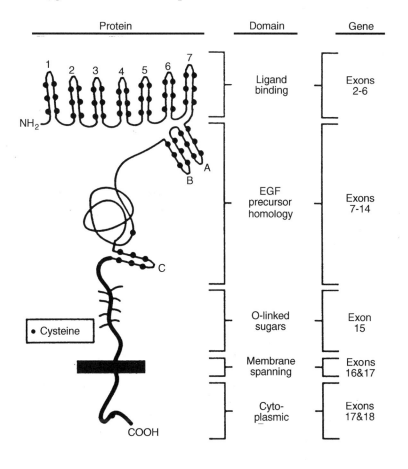

Figure 1.9
LDL receptor structure. The LDL receptor consists of 839 amino acids. The various receptor domains are shown together with the exons that code for them. Source: Hobbs *et al.* (1990) *Annual Review of Genetics* **24**, 133.

approximately 2.5 days in normals to 4.5 days in FH heterozygotes and 6 days in homozygotes. Non-receptor mediated removal of plasma LDL is not well understood.

High density lipoproteins

High density lipoproteins (HDL) are the smallest of the lipoprotein species and transport approximately 20–30% of plasma cholesterol. They are the most heterogeneous of the lipoproteins as many of their components are subject to rapid exchange with other lipoproteins and to modification by enzyme activity.

Nascent HDL in the form of bilayer discs containing apoprotein A and phospholipid is secreted by the liver and intestine. These transient particles rapidly become spherical as they take up free cholesterol from cell membranes and other lipoproteins and esterify it to cholesterol ester (which forms a lipid core to the particle) through the action of lecithin cholesterol acyl transferase (LCAT) enzyme. This enzyme circulates with HDL, and apoprotein A-I (the major HDL apoprotein) is important in its activation.

HDL is also modified by lipid exchange with lipoproteins of lower density. Cholesterol ester formed on HDL transfers to other lipoproteins via cholesterol ester transfer protein (CETP) in exchange for triglyceride.

Mature HDL consists of two principal subclasses, HDL_2 and HDL_3, and their respective concentrations are in part determined by the metabolism of triglyceride-rich lipoproteins. It is likely that the more dense HDL_3 is converted to HDL_2 by the acquisition of phospholipid and free cholesterol shed from VLDL and chylomicrons during their lipolysis. On the other hand the triglyceride-enriched HDL_2 may be converted back to HDL_3 through the action of hepatic lipase.

More recently, HDL particles have been subclassified according to whether they contain one or both of the principal HDL apoproteins, A-I and A-II. Whereas virtually all HDL particles contain A-I, not all contain A-II so that on the basis of apoprotein A composition particles are designated lipoprotein A-I (Lp A-I) or lipoprotein A-I/A-II (Lp A-I/A-II). The metabolism of these particles is likely to be different and further work is needed to delineate the pathways in detail. However, there is increasing evidence that Lp A-I containing particles, which predominate in HDL_2, are of particular importance in protecting against CHD.

Reverse cholesterol transport

HDL is involved in reverse cholesterol transport whereby cholesterol surplus to cellular requirements is returned from the periphery to the liver for

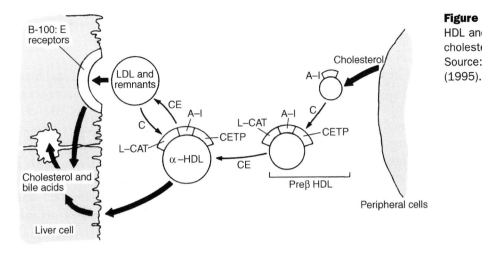

Figure 1.10
HDL and reverse cholesterol transport. Source: Havel and Kane (1995).

excretion (Figure 1.10). HDL can act as an acceptor for free cholesterol from tissues. The free cholesterol is esterified by the enzyme LCAT and enters the hydrophobic lipid-core of the particle.

There is accumulating evidence that a tiny fraction (accounting for approximately 5% of apoprotein A-I) of HDL, termed pre-beta HDL, is important as the acceptor of cellular free cholesterol. There is still a lot to learn concerning the interaction of pre-beta HDL with cells: it is not yet known whether a true receptor is involved but there is no doubt that the HDL/cell interaction stimulates a complex series of reactions which results in the translocation of free cholesterol from its storage form as cholesterol ester to the cell surface.

The cholesterol ester on HDL can return to the liver directly with subsequent recirculation of the particle. However, this process is quantitatively less important than the indirect transfer of HDL cholesterol ester to the liver. Cholesterol ester transfers from HDL to lipoproteins of lower density such as VLDL and LDL via CETP. Thus the major part of cholesterol ester formed within HDL returns to the liver in other lipoproteins.

Lipids, lipoproteins and atherogenesis

LDL cholesterol explains the link between plasma cholesterol, atherosclerosis and CHD. In recent years much has been learned about the interaction of this lipoprotein with cells important in atherogenesis. Essential insights have come from studies of non-human primates. These experiments have pointed to the important role of the monocyte macro-phage in the formation of foam cells which comprise the fatty streak – the initial lesion of atherosclerosis.

When experimental animals (including primates) are fed a high-fat, high-cholesterol diet, the first identifiable lesion is the adhesion of monocytes to arterial endothelium. At a later stage monocytes penetrate the endothelium, accumulate in the subendothelial space and acquire the characteristics of macrophages, which engulf lipid and become lipid-laden foam cells.

This process appears to be toxic to the overlying endothelium, which is disrupted. This allows platelet adhesion and aggregation with release of potent growth factors that stimulate smooth muscle proliferation and connective tissue accumulation, with consequent development of the ma-ture atherosclerotic plaque (Figure 1.11).

MODIFIED LDL

When the importance of the monocyte macrophage in foam cell formation was established, important experiments to study their interaction with LDL were performed. When incubated with native LDL, monocyte/macrophages did not accumulate lipid to any great extent and foam cells were not formed. This result was perhaps to be expected as the LDL receptor is protective in the sense that it is the major pathway by which LDL is cleared from the circulation by the liver. Further, patients with familial hyper-cholesterolaemia who lack functioning LDL receptors develop premature and extensive atherosclerosis.

In landmark experiments, Goldstein and Brown and colleagues showed that if LDL was chemically modified it was taken up avidly by monocyte/macrophages with foam cell formation (Brown and Goldstein, 1983). This process appeared to be receptor-mediated and the receptor was termed the scavenger receptor. A crucial difference between this receptor and the classical LDL receptor is its lack of down-regulation with increasing cellular cholesterol accumulation. Therefore by this process massive cholesterol accumulation can occur, resulting in lipid-laden foam cells.

Steinberg and colleagues showed that a likely *in vivo* modification of LDL resulting in uptake by monocyte/macrophages is peroxidation (Stein-berg *et al.*, 1989). Indeed oxidatively modified LDL may contribute to atherogenesis in other ways, including direct cytotoxicity to arterial endo-thelium and the stimulation of monocyte adhesion and monocyte chem-otaxis (Figure 1.12). Modified LDL may also interact with the coagulation system through increased expression of tissue factor (thromboplastin) and increased expression of plasminogen activator inhibitor I. These effects enhance the likelihood of activation of the coagulation cascade. Oxidized LDL may also have important effects on arterial tone through inhibition of

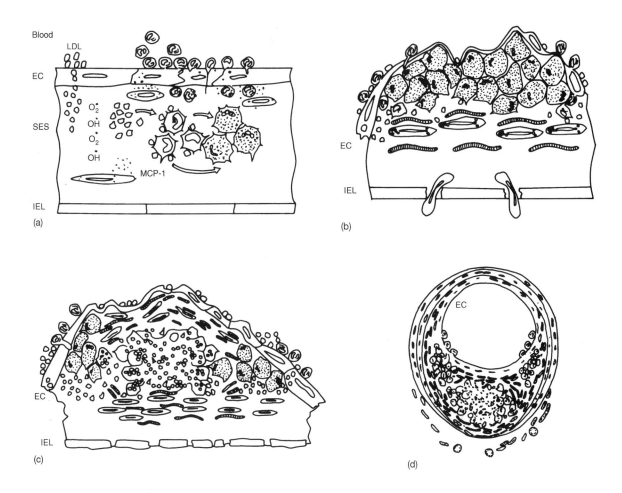

Key: EC endothelial cell; SES subendothelial space; IEL internal elastic lamina; LDL low density lipoprotein;MCP-1 monocyte chemotactic protein 1.

Figure 1.11 Development of atheroma.
(a) *Response-to-injury hypothesis: foam cell formation.* Plasma LDL crosses the endothelium and enters the SES. Here LDL is oxidatively modified by reactive oxygen spaces and is recognised by macrophage receptors. Blood monocytes attach to and penetrate through the endothelial barrier into the SES under the influence of MCP-1 and other factors. In the SES monocytes differentiate into macrophages, take up oxidatively-modified LDL and become foam cells. (b) *The fatty streak.* Continued monocyte recruitment, macrophage differentiation and LDL uptake lead to fatty streak formation. Smooth muscle cells migrate through the IEL and proliferate in response to mitogens such as platelet-derived growth factor. (c) *The transitional lesion.* The transitional lesion involves an intermediate lesion between the fatty streak and the established atherosclerotic plaque. Arterial wall thickness is increased but there is no lumen narrowing. The lesion is characterised by foam cell disruption and accumulation of extracellular lipid. Myointimal cells proliferate and synthesise connective tissue matrix. The internal elastic lamina fragments. (d) *The established lesion.* The lumen is narrowed by a mature fibrous plaque containing a lipid core of extracellular lipid and cholesterol crystals. Foam cells are prominent at the plaque edges and lymphocytes are present in the thickened intima. These plaques can rupture or erode triggering a platelet thrombus with consequent acute coronary syndromes.
Adapted from Schwartz, C.J. *et al.* (1991).

Figure 1.12
Oxidized LDL and
atherosclerosis.

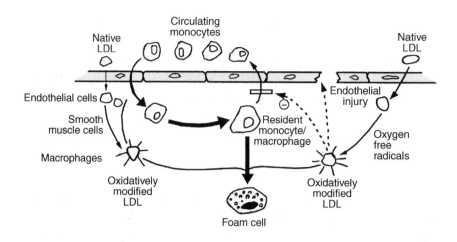

endothelium-derived relaxing factor and enhanced expression of endothelin, which is a potent vasoconstrictor.

Support for the concept of the atherogenicity of oxidatively modified LDL has come from studies in experimental atherosclerotic animals. In these experiments antioxidants have been shown to inhibit LDL modification, reduce LDL uptake into the arterial wall and protect against atherosclerosis. The clinical implications arising from knowledge of the importance of oxidatively modified LDL will become apparent when dietary therapy and the role of antioxidant supplements are discussed.

Figure 1.13
Low-density lipoprotein subfractions: distribution of human plasma LDL subclass density and particle size. * LDL subclass density profiles obtained by density gradient ultracentrifugation and representative of a typical normal, healthy female (– · · –), male (— ‾ —) and CAD patient (——). ** LDL particle size as determined by 2% to 16% gradient gel electrophorosis. Reproduced from Griffin, B.A. (1995) in *Dyslipidaemia* (ed. D.J. Betteridge) *Clin. Endocrinol. Metab.* **9**, 687–703.

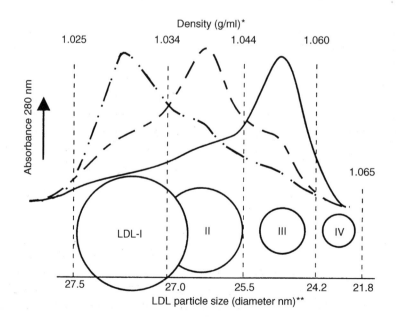

LDL SUBFRACTIONS

LDL is heterogeneous (Krauss and Burke, 1982) and can be separated on density gradient ultracentrifugation into subclasses that vary in size, density and lipid content (Figure 1.13). In healthy subjects the most abundant LDL subclass is LDL-II. Women have proportionately more of the larger, less dense LDL-I particles than men. Conversely, men have proportionately more of the smaller, denser LDL-III particles. LDL heterogeneity can also be assessed on gels where smaller, denser particles give rise to pattern B and larger, less dense particles to pattern A.

It is clear from the work of Austin and Krauss and others that LDL pattern B is strongly related to CHD risk (Austin *et al.*, 1988). This relationship remains to be fully explained but possible explanations include the slower fractional catabolic rate of dense LDL and its increased susceptibility to oxidation.

HDL AND PROTECTION FROM CHD

HDL cholesterol is inversely related to CHD risk, as discussed in detail in Part Two. The mechanisms by which increasing HDL concentrations are protective and low levels increase risk remain to be determined. The involvement of HDL in reverse cholesterol transport is an attractive explanation for its protective role but has not yet been proved. According to this hypothesis, the high levels of HDL would be associated with effective transport of cholesterol from peripheral tissues, including arterial wall, to the liver for excretion in bile or conversion to bile acids. An alternative hypothesis does not attach a specific protective role to HDL but suggests that the plasma HDL concentration reflects the efficiency or otherwise of the metabolism of triglyceride-rich lipoproteins, this process being directly related to atherogenesis.

Other potential ways by which HDL may protect against atherogenesis and CHD include inhibition of the oxidative modification of LDL lipid and protein. Effects of HDL on thrombotic tendency through inhibition of platelet aggregation and stimulation of the production of the potent platelet inhibitor and vasodilator, prostacyclin, from arterial endothelium may also be important.

TRIGLYCERIDES AND ATHEROGENESIS

Triglyceride accumulation is not a feature of the atherosclerotic plaque but triglyceride-rich lipoproteins also contain cholesterol esters and it is likely that some of these are directly atherogenic. There is little doubt that remnant particles fall into this category. It was Zilversmit who originally proposed that triglyceride-rich lipoproteins might be atherogenic and that the degree of postprandial lipoprotein metabolism may be central to atherogenesis (Zilversmit, 1979).

In the rare but important disease, Type III or dysbetalipoproteinaemia (discussed in detail in Chapter 5), there is marked accumulation of remnant particles and this is associated with premature extensive atherosclerosis not only in coronary but also in peripheral arteries. Laboratory studies have demonstrated that these lipoproteins can interact directly with monocyte/ macrophages to produce foam cells.

Hypertriglyceridaemia is associated with alterations in the metabolism of other lipoproteins which may explain its relationship to CHD risk. It is often inversely related to HDL such that as triglycerides increase, HDL cholesterol concentrations decrease.

Triglycerides are also related to alterations in the distribution of LDL subclasses. In hypertriglyceridaemic individuals there is a preponderance of small, dense LDL particles. As discussed earlier, there is evidence that these particles are highly atherogenic. It has been calculated that the plasma triglyceride concentration accounts for much of the variability in LDL subfraction distribution. This relationship can be explained by the lipid exchange promoted by hypertriglyceridaemia together with the action of hepatic lipase. Triglyceride exchanges for cholesterol ester via CETP to LDL, and triglyceride-rich LDL is a substrate for hepatic lipase resulting in the formation of lipid-poor, protein-rich LDL particles.

A further explanation for the link between plasma triglyceride and CHD risk relates to the association between hypertriglyceridaemia and coagulation factors. Factor VII is an important component of the extrinsic coagulation system and in prospective studies has been shown to be an independent predictor of CHD. Increasing plasma triglycerides are positively correlated with the activity of factor VII and some of the day-to-day variation in factor VII coagulation activity is related to dietary fat intake.

Plasma triglyceride concentration is also positively correlated with activity of plasminogen activator inhibitor 1 (PAI-1). PAI-1 is an inhibitor of plasminogen activation and has been shown to be increased in young myocardial infarction patients.

LIPOPROTEIN(A)

There is considerable current interest in this lipoprotein, which consists of LDL with an additional apoprotein – apoprotein(a) – attached to it via a disulphide bond (Figure 1.14). Apoprotein(a) has striking structural homology with plasminogen, a zymogen of the coagulation and fibrinolytic system.

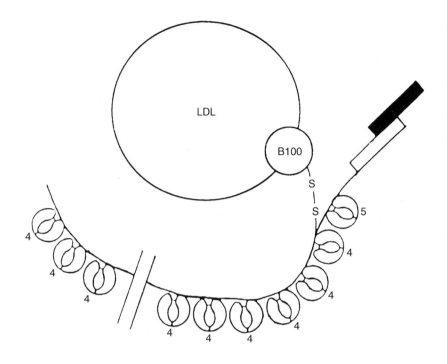

Figure 1.14
Lipoprotein(a).
Lipoprotein(a) consists of
LDL joined by a single
disulphide bridge to
apoprotein (a), which
consists of the protease
domain, kringle 5 and a
variable number of kringle
4 repeats of plasminogen.
Source: Scanu, A.M.
(1990) Lipoprotein(a), in
*Ballière's Clinical
Endocrinology and
Metabolism: Lipid and
Lipoprotein Disorders* (ed.
D.J. Betteridge), Vol. 4,
No. 4.

Lipoprotein(a) concentrations vary widely within and between populations. In Europeans most individuals have low levels but there is a pronounced positive skew to the distribution with very high levels in some people. This variation appears to be largely determined by the apoprotein(a) gene locus. Plasma concentrations correlate inversely with the molecular mass of apoprotein(a), which exists in many different size polymorphisms.

The physiology of lipoprotein(a) remains poorly understood but its rate of production appears to be a major determinant of its plasma concentration. It is likely that apoprotein(a) is directly secreted by the liver and then associates with LDL.

The importance of lipoprotein(a) relates to its association with CHD risk and, from its structural homology with plasminogen, it is tempting to speculate that this lipoprotein may be an important link with the coagulation system. Many case control studies have demonstrated that high lipoprotein(a) concentrations relate to CHD risk but the association appears to be influenced by the prevailing LDL concentration – the higher the LDL, the stronger the relationship between lipoprotein(a) and CHD. Lipoprotein(a) also appears to be a risk factor for restenosis after angioplasty and coronary artery bypass grafting and for accelerated coronary disease in cardiac transplant patients. In patients with familial hypercholesterolaemia and CHD, lipoprotein(a) concentrations are increased compared with those without CHD. Lipoprotein(a) has also been demonstrated in atheromatous lesions.

Some recent prospective studies have failed to demonstrate an association between lipoprotein(a) and CHD and these findings have cast doubt on the importance of lipoprotein(a) as an independent risk factor. The authors' current opinion is that lipoprotein(a) is of importance in the presence of high LDL concentrations. Whether the pathogenetic role of lipoprotein(a) depends on its homology with plasminogen and possible interference with normal fibrinolysis remains to be determined.

The 'candidate' plaque for clinical events

Detailed histopathological examination of coronary arteries from subjects dying of acute myocardial infarction has revealed that in the great majority of cases the lesion precipitating coronary occlusion is plaque fissuring, allowing intraplaque haemorrhage and platelet thrombosis (Davies and Thomas, 1981; Davies, 1996). This is the basis for the use of platelet active agents and antithrombolytic therapy in acute myocardial infarction. From studies such as these it has become clear that the plaques most likely to trigger an event – the so-called candidate lesions – are lipid-rich with a relatively thin fibrous cap laden with foam cells. These lesions, which represent only a small proportion of total plaques, are often not associated with a large degree of stenosis – about 30–50% (Plate 1).

Epidemiology

2

Historical perspective

The roots of epidemiological investigation extend back to the early eighteenth century. In 1727 Brunner, conducting his father-in-law's autopsy, described the atherosclerotic aorta as 'ruptured, lacerated and rotten, like fruit'. In 1755 Albrecht von Haller passed comment on another post-mortem specimen. Opening into the aortic plaques, he found a yellow mush between the muscular fibres and the intima which was soft and pultaceous. Since Greek times, the word atheroma had been used to describe any closed sac filled with a porridge-like material (*athere* means mush or gruel) and he likened the plaques to 'atheromata'. He also noted that the same aorta had harder and drier plaques (more fibrotic) and inferred that a gradual process of hardening took place, eventually culminating in a hard, bone-like structure. John Hunter's own post-mortem in 1793 at St George's Hospital revealed vascular tissue covered with an 'exudation of coagulating lymph' and the coronary arteries were said to 'ramify through the substance of the heart in the state of bony tubes'.

Cholesterol was first described in the eighteenth century, having been cystallized from alcoholic extracts of gallstones. In 1816 it was named from the Greek *chole* (bile) and *steros* (solid). Its presence in blood was demonstrated in 1838 and in 1843 Vogel showed that it was present in atherosclerotic plaques. As happened so often in the early epidemiology of heart disease, the finding received little attention.

The advent of systematic cell microscopy in the second half of the nineteenth century elucidated the morphological characteristics of the atheromatous plaque, confirming the deposition of free and esterified cholesterol as the hallmark lesion. By the early twentieth century, study of several diseases – hypothyroidism, nephrotic syndrome and what became later identified as familial hypercholesterolaemia – showed that premature severe atherosclerosis was linked to the level of cholesterol.

Following the first description of acute myocardial infarction in 1910, it soon became known that people recovering from myocardial infarction had higher mean serum cholesterol levels than controls. By the 1930s, it was evident that the modern epidemic of coronary heart disease was under way, a scourge that few industrialized countries have been able to escape.

Once it was realized in the early twentieth century that geographical differences in the frequency of coronary heart disease existed, 'geographical pathology' became a respectable research interest. Initially, differences between populations were identified largely by European investigators working in the colonies and many studies linked low dietary fat intake with a low level of atherosclerosis. Conversely, in 1925 Kuczynski studied Asian Kirghiz plainsmen and correlated their diet rich in meat and milk to their excessive prevalence of obesity, arcus senilis and premature atherosclerosis.

In 1916 DeLangen, a physician from Utrecht, showed that Indonesian nationals had lower levels of blood cholesterol than their Dutch counterparts and he related this to the increased incidence of atherosclerosis in the Netherlands. His significant observation was that Indonesian stewards on Dutch passenger ships eating Dutch food had levels similar to those found in the Netherlands. Unfortunately, this forerunner of later important migration studies was published in a Dutch language journal and passed unnoticed.

After the great depression and World War II, there was an explosion of interest in 'geographical pathology' when it was discovered that in countries such as the United States, Finland and in much of northern Europe, atherosclerotic disease accounted for more than half the total mortality.

America was further shocked in 1953 when Major William Enos examined the coronary arteries of 300 soldiers (mean age 22.1 years) killed in action in the Korean War. Only 25% were free of visible atherosclerotic lesions, in complete contrast to their Korean counterparts. This should have been no surprise as in 1915 Monckeberg had drawn similar conclusions from German troops killed in World War I – again a piece of research that failed to surface. In contrast, some countries such as Japan, those bordering the Mediterranean and most of the under-developed world were enjoying much lower rates of coronary mortality and the search was on to identify individual risk factors to explain these differences.

Ancel Keys, a nutritional physiologist from Minnesota became the dominant figure through the 1950s and 1960s as his high-quality research began to establish the cholesterol hypothesis. With the development of the risk factor concept in 1961 there evolved a predictive capacity for coronary heart disease unparalleled in almost any other condition. Many studies began to tell the same story with the major risk factors of hypercholesterolaemia, high blood pressure and smoking coming to the fore and with hypercholesterolaemia assuming a pivotal central role. Quantitative estimates of how much coronary disease can be accounted for by each risk factor became possible and with them the beginnings of opportunities for effective prevention.

Cardiovascular death

About a quarter of all deaths world-wide are caused by cardiovascular diseases (mostly CHD and strokes). In developed countries, about 50% of deaths are due to cardiovascular disease whereas in developing countries the proportion is only about 15%. However, as 80% of the world's deaths occur in developing countries, the total number of cardiovascular deaths is roughly equally divided between developed and developing nations.

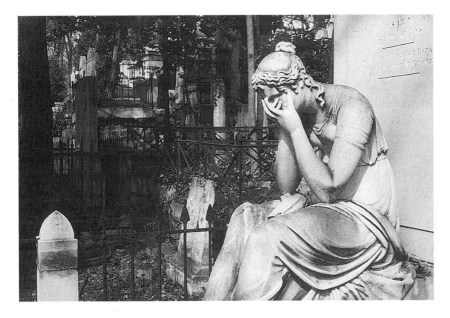

In the same way that CHD mortality rates show international variation, so too do deaths from other cardiovascular causes. Stroke is a leading cause of death in China, cardiomyopathies and hypertensive heart disease in Africa and in many countries rheumatic heart disease remains common.

Table 2.1 shows the number of CHD deaths for each cerebrovascular death in males (1985–1989). This clearly shows that different risk factors or different levels of similar risk factors are at work around the world. In essence, this is reflected by the central importance of dyslipidaemia in the development of CHD and the importance of hypertension in the aetiology of stroke.

Table 2.1
Number of CHD deaths for each cerebrovascular death in males, 1985–1989

Country	No. deaths
USA	4.63
New Zealand	4.19
Australia	3.61
England and Wales	3.58
Singapore	2.20
Sri Lanka	1.94
France	1.44
Hong Kong	0.91
Japan	0.46
Korea	0.08

THE POSITION IN THE UK

As in the rest of the developed world, cardiovascular disease remains the leading cause of death in the UK (Figure 2.1): 26% of all deaths are caused by CHD, 61% by the acute myocardial infarction (and thereby the victims are prevented from receiving secondary prevention benefits). There are sex differences, males being affected not only more often but at an earlier age.

In Figure 2.1 some cardiovascular causes of death (e.g. other cardiac problems, peripheral vascular disease) are included in 'other diseases'.

UK CHD factsheet

- Cardiovascular disease is the main cause of death in the UK, accounting for nearly 300 000 deaths per year.
- Coronary heart disease by itself is the single largest cause of death: nearly 170 000 people died from CHD in 1992. This represents nearly 500 deaths/day (a daily Jumbo Jet disaster) or 8 deaths/GP per year.
- One in three men die from CHD.
- One in four women die from CHD.
- CHD is the major cause of premature death in both sexes (5000 males under 55). This rate is twice that of many other western countries.
- CHD is also responsible for considerable morbidity:
  - 330 000 people have a heart attack each year;
  - 1.9 million have angina;
  - 0.5 million suffer from heart failure.
- Death rates (Figure 2.2) have been falling since the late 1970s:
  - in England and Wales by 22% for men aged 35–74 (1979–1989) and by 15% for women
  - in Scotland by 19% and 14%, respectively
  - in Northern Ireland by 20% and 18%, respectively

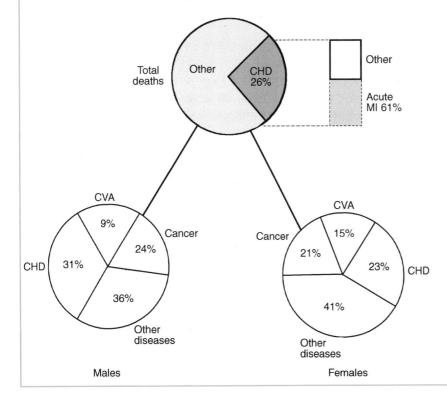

Figure 2.1
Causes of death in UK: differences between males and females. Note that some cardiovascular causes (e.g. other cardiac problems, peripheral vascular disease) are included in the category 'other diseases'. CHD = coronary heart disease; CVA = cardiovascular accident; MI = myocardial infarction.

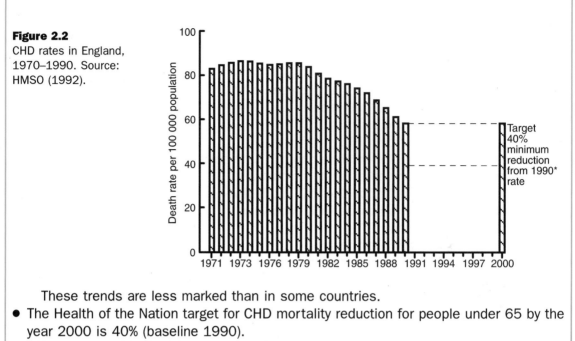

Figure 2.2
CHD rates in England, 1970–1990. Source: HMSO (1992).

These trends are less marked than in some countries.

- The Health of the Nation target for CHD mortality reduction for people under 65 by the year 2000 is 40% (baseline 1990).
- CHD cost the NHS £1.42 billion in 1994:
  - hospital costs 45%
  - medicines 35%
  - GP/community/ambulance 19%

  Only 1% is spent on health promotion.
- The 53 million working days lost due to CHD (10% of all sickness absence) cost £463 million in invalidity benefit and an estimated £3 billion in lost production.

Studies between populations

THE SEVEN COUNTRIES STUDY

In 1980 Ancel Keys published his analysis of CHD in 12 763 middle-aged men divided into 16 cohorts within the seven countries Japan, Italy, Greece, the Netherlands, Yugoslavia, Finland and the United States. These countries were deliberately chosen because they were known to have differing prevalence rates for CHD death. Initially, five and ten-year follow-up data were collected but such was the significance of the study that survivors are still being studied and important reports are still being produced.

There were three major findings:

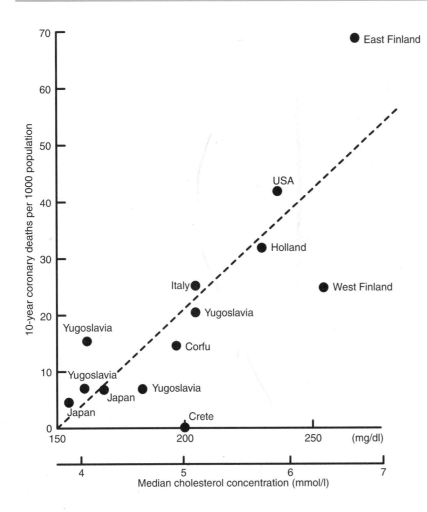

Figure 2.3
Relationship between median plasma cholesterol level and 10-year CHD mortality in 16 male cohorts of the Seven Countries Study. Source: Keys (1980).

1. The mean serum total cholesterol concentration in a community is directly related to that community's CHD mortality (Figure 2.3). East Finland recorded the highest mean serum total cholesterol at 6.6 mmol/l and had CHD mortality rates more than 15 times those of Ushibaka in Japan where the mean serum total cholesterol was 4.1 mmol/l.
2. The mean serum total cholesterol concentration in a community (and by inference, therefore, the CHD mortality) is directly related to the saturated fat content in the usual diet of that community (Figure 2.4).
3. The mean serum total cholesterol concentration is the key factor in determining a community's risk of CHD. The effect of hypertension, smoking, diabetes and lack of exercise was only additional when the coronary arteries were susceptible because of hypercholesterolaemia. Communities with low mean serum total cholesterol levels had low rates of CHD despite high levels of other risk factors (e.g. Japan).

Figure 2.4
Relationship between
blood cholesterol and
saturated fat intake in diet
in the Seven Countries
Study. Source: Keys
(1980).

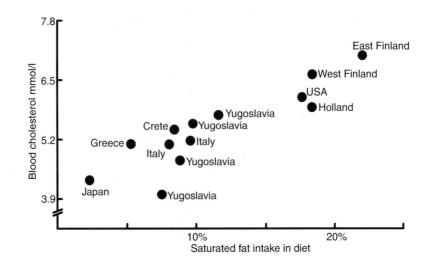

A number of international comparative studies have since found similar associations. In 1986 Simons presented data from 19 countries indicating the same relationship for serum cholesterol and CHD death.

CURRENT INTERNATIONAL DIFFERENCES

Figure 2.5 shows CHD mortality rates for men and women in the industrialized world. There are marked contrasts in the rates for northern and eastern European countries and those of the Mediterranean countries and Japan. The differences can be understood in terms of life style (in essence dietary and smoking habits) and socio-economic factors. That they are not due to in-built genetic factors is demonstrated by studies of migrants.

The Ni Hon San Study, 1977

Despite high levels of smoking and hypertension, the natural population of Japan has a low rate of CHD. The Ni Hon San study (Table 2.2) followed migrants from Japan (**Nippon**) to Hawaii (**Honolulu**) and California (**San** Francisco). Although rates of hypertension and smoking fell, mean total serum cholesterol rose and with it the CHD rate.

As a change in gene structure over such a short period of time is untenable, the differences must have been brought about by environmental change, namely the assimilation of an increasingly westernized diet.

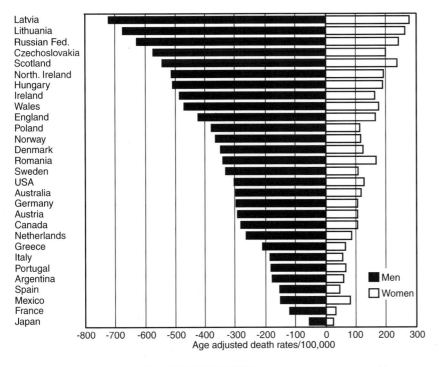

Figure 2.5
CHD death rates for men and women aged 35–74 in selected industrialized countries, 1991. Source: as Figure 2.6

CHD AND ECONOMIC DEVELOPMENT

International comparisons (Figure 2.5), like other 'league tables', are not static but dynamic and countries shift their positions as their CHD rates alter (Figure 2.6).

- CHD rates are falling in the wealthy countries of Europe and in the United States and Australasia. The rates of fall vary, however. For example, between 1970 and 1985 they fell by 48% in the United States, but by only 11% in England over the same period.
- CHD rates are rising in many countries of central and eastern Europe and the Russian Federation (the old 'Iron Curtain' is becoming the 'Coronary Curtain').

Factor	Japan	Honolulu	San Francisco
Acute MI rate/1000	7.3	13.2	31.4
Hypertensive heart disease/ 1000	9.3	1.4	4.6
Non-smokers (%)	26.0	57.0	64.0
Mean serum total cholesterol (mmol/l)	4.7	5.6	5.9

Table 2.2
Ni Hon San study (1977) of migrants from Japan to Hawaii and California

Figure 2.6
Reductions in CHD death rates for men and women aged 35–74 in selected countries, between 1981 and 1991. Source: Boaz, Kaduskar and Rayner (1996) *Coronary Heart Disease Statistics*, Figs 1.11a, b, British Heart Foundation.

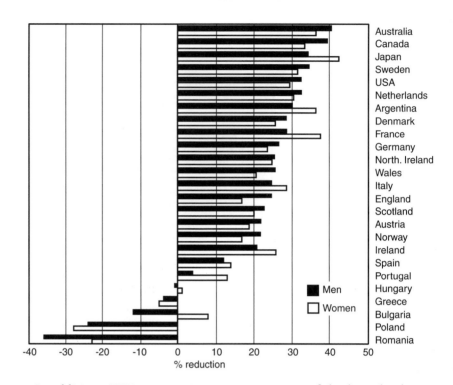

- In addition, CHD is emerging as a major cause of death in developing countries.

A pattern has emerged of rising CHD with increasing economic development (industrialization, 'westernization'). Once they have become mature, industrialized countries then show reducing levels. In 1921 the number of CHD and cancer deaths in the UK equalled those from infectious disease. Within 10 years, cardiovascular diseases were pre-eminent as increasing prosperity reduced the incidence of deaths from infection. This is mirrored in Latin America at present where, over the next 25 years, deaths from cardiovascular disease are expected to number five times those from infectious and parasitic disease compared with roughly equal numbers in the two groups in 1985.

Privotal to these changes is the adoption of a 'rich' western diet, with its relationships to raised serum cholesterol and hypertension. With a 'rich' diet the secondary role of smoking in the aetiology of atherosclerotic disease becomes manifest on a large scale. 'Rich' diet is high in total fat (especially saturated fat), high in cholesterol, sugar, salt, alcohol and unnecessary calories and low in potassium, fibre and other essential nutrients. With a lower level of energy expenditure resulting from the use of the car, the television and automated labour, the 'couch potato' is born.

MONICA is an ongoing WHO programme for MONItoring trends and determinants in CArdiovascular disease in 26 countries. Comparative mean serum cholesterol levels between countries are broadly in line with CHD trends:

China 4.1 mmol/l
United States 5.3 mmol/l
Scotland 6.2 mmol/l
Czechoslovakia 6.3 mmol/l

In general, countries with mean serum cholesterol levels lower than 4.5–5.0 mmol/l seem to have little CHD.

THREE COUNTRIES IN FOCUS: UNITED STATES, JAPAN AND HUNGARY

In the **United States**, CHD rates have approximately halved in the last two decades. Most of this fall results from the improved risk factor status of the population (Figure 2.7). Consumption of total fat, saturated fat, cholesterol, salt and cigarettes has fallen whereas consumption of polyunsaturates, fish and fibre and the partaking of exercise have risen. Surprisingly, as in the UK, mean body weight has risen.

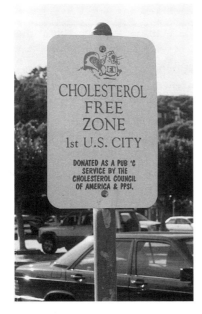

Figure 2.7
Signpost in Sausolito, California.

In the 1980s, a national system for monitoring CHD trends was established and in 1988 the National Cholesterol Education Programme recommended the testing of all adults every five years and issued guidelines to physicians. The 'Know your Number' campaign was launched and by

Figure 2.8
Differential price rises in Hungary. Source: Kaposvari and Bales (1988), *Mag yarovszag*, Feb. 26.

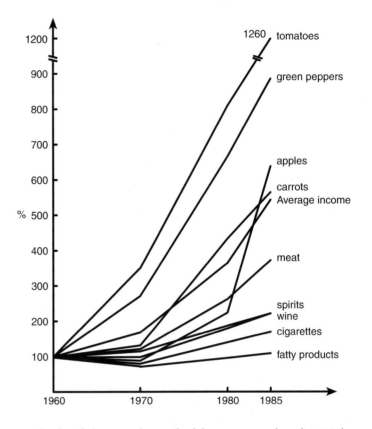

1989 two-thirds of the population had been screened and 25% knew the result. The 1980s also saw a five-fold increase in the prescribing of lipid lowering drugs and a nine-fold increase in CHD prevention consultations. Mean cholesterol levels dropped by 3–4%.

Japan has proved the exception, so far, to the 'industrialization' pattern. Although two-thirds of Japanese men smoke and there are high levels of hypertension, CHD rates have been amongst the lowest in the world. This is attributed to low saturated fat in the diet and low mean serum cholesterol (cf. the Seven Countries Study). Despite an already low mortality, the rates of further improvement have been amongst the highest in the world. This probably relates to improved detection and management of hypertension and a reduction of dietary sodium rather than further changes in lipid factors. Indeed, there is some evidence for adverse change in saturated fat consumption and the future may see a deterioration in circumstances.

Evidence from eastern Europe and Russia to explain their countries' dramatic rise in CHD rates is very scarce. From **Hungary** comes intriguing evidence that economic factors can influence a nation's dietary habits. Differential price rises favour lifestyle habits that may be responsible for higher levels of CHD (Figure 2.8).

The French paradox

The low rates of CHD in France are not explained by an analysis of standard risk factors alone. Nationalistic scepticism has at various stages suggested the French must somehow 'cook the books' but the MONICA study reveals this theory to be wrong. The comparison to a high risk country such as Scotland is interesting (Table 2.3).

Risk factor	Scotland	France
CHD mortality/100 000 (40–69 y)	540	120
Mean serum cholesterol (mmol/l)	6.3	5.8
Systolic pressure (mm Hg)	138	139
Smokers (%)	52	36
HDL cholesterol	1.34	1.34

Table 2.3
Risk factors and CHD mortality in Scotland and France

Whilst there are fewer smokers in France, it is in the area of diet that significant changes appear. The 'Mediterranean diet' incorporates increased fruit and vegetable intake, higher mono- and polyunsaturated fatty acid levels and reduced saturated fats. There is increased soluble and insoluble fibre, a dash of garlic and, of course, the wine. There is evidence for better nutrition generally in wine-drinking countries and again the comparison with Scotland is valid (Table 2.4).

Substance	Scotland	France
Vegetables (g/day)	114 (12% nil)	260
Fruit (g/day)	70 (20% nil)	180
Monounsaturated fat intake	Low	High
Wine intake	Low	High

Table 2.4
Nutrition and wine intake in Scotland and France

France not only leads the world in wine consumption but also has the highest per capita overall alcohol intake. The consumption of any alcohol is inversely related to CHD. The benefit extends to up to 4–5 units/day and probably exerts its effect via increased HDL cholesterol production as well as anti-thrombotic effects on fibrinogen and platelet aggregation. The amount of ethanol itself may therefore be the active factor. It should be noted, however, that consumption in excess of 2 units/day increases mortality from other causes and higher levels of drinking are not recommended.

There is a suggestion that wine ethanol (particularly in red wine) may be the active factor and the search is on for a non-ethanol substance. Leading candidates include procyanidins, especially phytoalexins (antifungals found in grape skins with powerful anti-oxidant properties). As the skins persist for longer in the preparation of red wine, this may be significant.

Despite low levels of CHD in France, it is interesting to compare levels of screening and expenditure on lipid lowering agents with the UK (Table 2.5).

Table 2.5
Levels of screening and expenditure on lipid-lowering agents in France and UK

Country	Population (millions)	Percentage screened	Quarterly spending (1992)
France	56	65	£50 m
UK	56	17	£6.5 m

Studies within populations

The frequency distribution of cholesterol within a population, like many biological variables, is almost Gaussian with a slight positive skew (Figure 2.9). There are slight differences between men and women, younger women tending to have lower levels of serum cholesterol. The level tends to rise in men until their 40s and then flattens off, whereas in women the rise is maintained (Figure 2.10).

STUDIES IN THE UNITED STATES

Framingham
Data collection in this small town 18 miles west of Boston began with 740 volunteers in 1948. Eventually 5000 volunteers were amassed from the town's very stable 28 000 population and research is ongoing. Much of our understanding of the multifactional aetiology of CHD stems from this data and multivariate statistical analysis has helped to determine the net and joint effects of each risk factor.

The major findings establish a list of CHD risk factors that act in both sexes and at all ages but with different strengths:

1. Total cholesterol (TC) positively related to CHD.
2. LDL cholesterol, positively related to CHD.

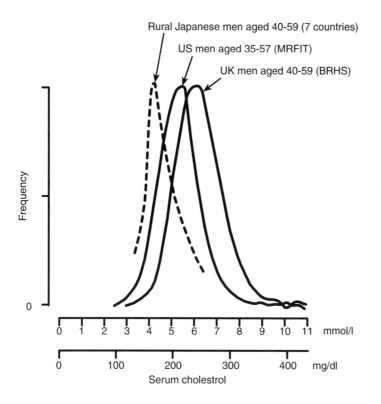

Rural Japanese men aged 40-59 (7 countries)

US men aged 35-57 (MRFIT)

UK men aged 40-59 (BRHS)

Figure 2.9
Serum cholesterol
distribution curves.
Source: Durrington (1989)
*Hyperlipidaemia –
Diagnosis and
Management*, Wright.

3. HDL cholesterol, inversely related to CHD. The ratio TC : HDL is established as an efficient lipid risk predictor (better than LDL : HDL). Although pivotal to Framingham data and in widespread use, the concept of ratios is debated. For example, in Japan, where both total cholesterol and HDL levels are low, calculated ratios are high but of course CHD incidence is low.

4. Hypertension. Systolic and disastolic pressures are equally good predictors; LVH is also a good predictor.

5. Smoking.

6. Diabetes and impaired glucose tolerance. Low HDL in female diabetics completely eliminates the normal female/male variation.

7. Lack of exercise.

8. Fibrinogen.

9. Alcohol intake – moderate intake is protective, excess increases risk.

10. Type A behaviour.

11. Family history – 30% increased risk if a parent died before age 65.

The quantification and interaction of risk associated with combinations of smoking, hypertension and hypercholesterolaemia is shown in Figure 2.11. Framingham data show that all cardiovascular risk factors contribute

Figure 2.10
Trends in lipoprotein levels in men and women according to age. Source: Kannel, W.B. (1988) *Nutrition Review* **46**, 66–78.

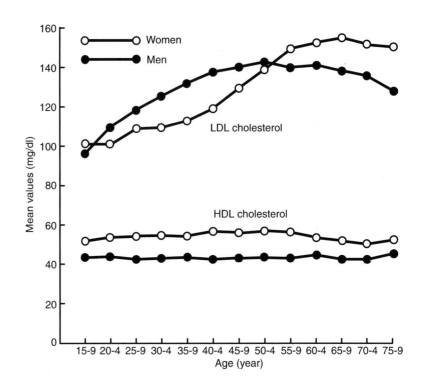

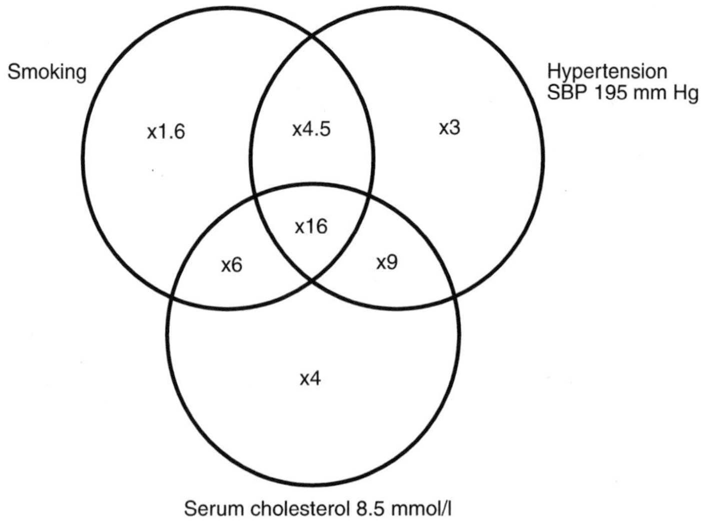

Figure 2.11
Quantification and interaction of risk associated with combinations of smoking, hypertension and hypercholesterolaemia.

to CHD and confirm the central role of dyslipidaemia. For cerebrovascular disease, hypertension predominates and lipids play a lesser role. For peripheral vascular disease, smoking and diabetes are paramount.

The Multiple Risk Factor Intervention Trial – MRFIT

Inspired by the findings of the Seven Countries Study, MRFIT was designed as a flagship trial to see if risk factor modification, especially dietary change and smoking reduction, would reduce CHD events. As a trial, the study was unsuccessful: there were no statistically significant differences between the usual care and intervention groups. The trial was conducted at a time of rising population awareness of CHD risk factors and it proved impossible to curtail the activities of the usual care group, who ceased to remain a genuine control population.

In total, 361 662 men aged 35–37 from 18 US cities were screened between 1973 and 1975. Data on 356 222 men followed up for six years was published in 1986 and 12-year data are now available. The value of the study is in its statistical precision, for at 70 times the size of the Framingham database the conclusions are very powerful (Figure 2.12).

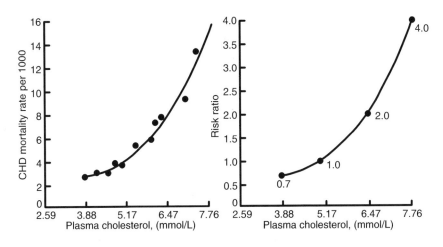

Figure 2.12
Relationship between total cholesterol concentration and coronary mortality in the Multiple Risk Factor Intervention Trial (MRFIT). Source: Grundy (1986) *JAMA* **256**, 2849–2858.

MRFIT revealed that the relationship between CHD and cholesterol was continuous, strong and graded across the range of cholesterol. There is no threshold level below which CHD events do not occur but the risk increases dramatically from a cholesterol level of about 5.2 mmol/l. MRFIT also reaffirmed the multiplicative effect of the major risk factors. At any level of a given risk factor, the coincidence of other factors increased the CHD risk. As only 3% of the study population were non-smokers with systolic BP < 118 mm Hg and total cholesterol < 4.7 mmol/l, the major risk factors are relevant to virtually the whole population of American males. The absolute risk of CHD for the lowest 3% was 3.09 per 10 000 person years, and for the group at highest risk it was 62.11 per 10 000 person years. This 20-fold increase corresponds to 684.6 excess deaths per 10 000 men for 11.6 years of follow-up.

British regional heart study (BRHS)

Regional differences in the UK, with a pronounced north/south divide, have been known for some time (Figure 2.13). The BRHS was designed to determine the personal and environmental risk factors active in the UK and whether they would explain the geographical variation in CHD mortality.

Between 1978 and 1980, 7735 men aged 40–59, randomly chosen from general practices in 24 towns in England, Scotland and Wales, were examined. After 4.2 years of follow-up, there had been 202 cases of major CHD and it is interesting to note that 197 of these had either raised cholesterol or high blood pressure or were smokers.

There were three main areas of data collection:

Figure 2.13
CHD: regional differences (UK, annual death rates). Source: *Cardiovascular disease*, OPCS.

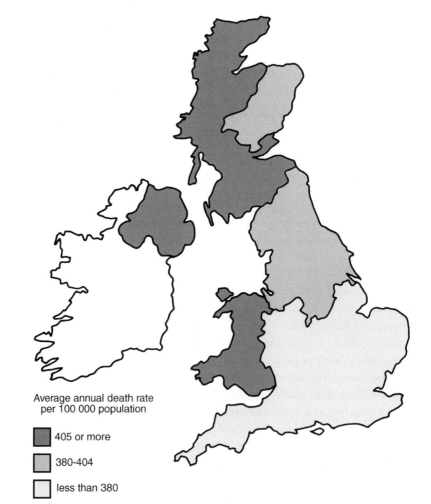

Average annual death rate
per 100 000 population

405 or more

380-404

less than 380

1. **Prevalence of CHD**

   ECG findings and a questionnaire established that 25% of the study population had evidence of CHD and the prevalence correlated well with local mortality rates. Even in the lowest age group (40–44 years) prevalence was 1 in 6.

2. **Personal risk factors**

   Each risk factor was divided into quintiles (fifths) with approximately 1500 men in each. The top and bottom quintiles were compared to produce a figure of relative risk. (Table 2.6). The predictive capacity of this data led to the development of a GP scoring system (the Shaper Score – Chapter 6).

Factor	Relative risk	Comment
Age	4.7	Even the middle quintile, the 'Average Man', had × 2 risk
Total cholesterol (TC)	3.1	
Low HDL	2.0	
Triglyceride (TG)		Association disappeared when adjusted for TC and HDL
Systolic BP	3.0	
Diastolic BP	3.1	
'Smoking years'	5.1	Smokers : non-smokers 3.0
Body mass index (BMI)	1.8	Association disappeared when adjusted for TC, HDL, TG, BP
Alcohol		No association

Table 2.6
Coronary risk factors in the British Regional Heart Study

Fifteen-year follow-up of 7142 initially healthy men now shows that a non-smoking, low BMI, physically active 50-year-old man has an 88% chance of living to 65. In contrast an obese, inactive smoker's chance is reduced to only 30%.

3. **Regional influences**

   It was found that mean serum total cholesterol levels were fairly constant across the 24 towns (6.0–6.6 mmol/l) and that there was no correlation with regional differences. It is important to note that this mean level is high and therefore the cholesterol factor is active right across the UK. In contrast, smoking and BP levels did vary, in keeping with geographical and social class differences.

Social class differences in the UK

Social class differences are a manifestation of the socio-economic forces at work in CHD causation (Figure 2.14). Sixty years ago CHD was more

Figure 2.14
CHD: social class differences. SMR = standardized mortality ratio. Source: OPCS (1986)

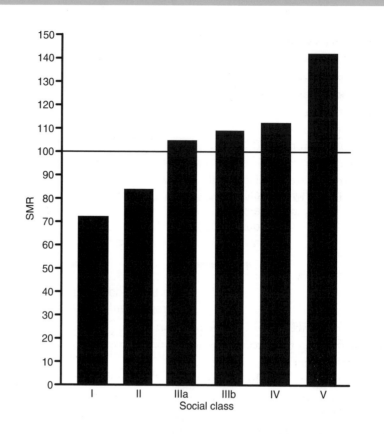

Table 2.7
Smoking and obesity trends in UK by social class

Factor		Social class			
		I II	IIIa	IIIb	IV V
Smoking (%)	M	22	27	36	**41**
	F	21	28	32	34
Obesity (%)	M	12	10	11	18
	F	11	13	18	**23**

common in social classes I and II but there has been a complete reversal, with the cross-over at some stage in the 1950s. The decline in CHD in social classes I and II almost completely accounts for the recent decline in CHD seen in the UK, there being no change in the rates for manual occupations.

Whilst serum cholesterol levels are highest in social class I and lowest in V, levels of blood pressure, smoking, fibrinogen and obesity show the reverse trend (Table 2.7). Unemployment has an increased relative risk of 3.56.

Clearly, important interventions could be targeted at obese social class IV/V women and class IV/V male smokers.

Immigrant populations in the UK

It became apparent from increased reports in the 1950s that there were large differences in CHD rates between immigrant populations (now over 1.5 million people) and UK nationals (Table 2.8).

1979–1983	Country of birth	Standardized mortality ratio (SMR) (England + Wales = 100)	
		Men	Women
CHD mortality	Scotland	111	119
	Ireland	114	120
	South Asia	136	146
	Caribbean	45	76
CVA mortality	Caribbean	176	210

Table 2.8
Mortality rates in immigrant populations aged 20–69 years in UK

For Afro-Caribbeans, the danger of stroke is greater than the risk of CHD and relates to increased prevalence of hypertension in both sexes and obesity in women.

For immigrants from India, Pakistan and Bangladesh, there are high rates of CHD and this finding is duplicated in other countries. There are very few data from South Asia itself but two studies suggest a low prevalence of CHD in rural India. In two North Indian cities, the prevalence of CHD judged by ECG changes showed rates equivalent to those in the UK.

The increased risk of South Asian immigrants is not explained in terms of standard risk factors. Furthermore, the increased risk also applies to second generation immigrants:

- Hindus from Gujurat in western India are vegetarian and have low levels of cholesterol, whereas Sikhs from the Punjab in North India and Muslims from Pakistan and Bangladesh have average levels.
- Blood pressure is average in Gujuratis, increased in Punjabis and reduced in Muslims.
- Smoking is low in Sikhs and all South Asian women, and average in Hindus and Muslims.

There were clues in a 1988 study of Bangladeshi migrants to East London, where a high prevalence of non-insulin dependent diabetes mellitus (NIDDM) was found. This was confirmed in the 1991 Southall study (McKeigue), which revealed the findings shown in Table 2.9.

The aggregation of diabetes, low HDL, high triglyceride, hypertension, central distribution of body fat and high levels of insulin is known as the **insulin resistance syndrome**, described by Reaven, and it is very likely that

Table 2.9
Southall study, 1991: risk factors in Europeans and South Asians

Risk factor	European	South Asian
Mean BP	121/78	126/82
BMI	25.9	25.7
Total cholesterol (mmol/l)	6.11	5.98
Diabetes (%)	4.8	19.6
Waist hip ratio	0.94	0.98
HDL	1.25	1.16
TG	1.48	1.73
Fasting insulin (mU/l)	7.2	9.8

some sort of genetic predisposition to develop insulin resistance exists in this group.

Similar findings have been described in New Zealand Maoris and Australian Aborigines consuming a western diet. The failure of insulin to suppress non-esterified fatty acids from adipose tissue may increase VLDL triglyceride, which may reduce HDL and produce smaller, more atherogenic LDL. This may have been a mechanism to use triglyceride rather than glucose as fuel at times of deprivation. This 'thrifty genotype' interacting with 'rich' western diet, together with traditional foods rich in saturates such as ghee, may be the explanation for the increased susceptibility to CHD.

Unfortunately, when adjusted for all features of the insulin resistance syndrome there is still an excess mortality in the South Asian group. Levels of exercise are also low in South Asian immigrants and the effect of modifying this should be evaluated.

STUDIES IN OTHER COUNTRIES

Many other intrapopulation studies confirm the establishment of serum cholesterol as the major risk factor for CHD. Earlier studies concentrated on establishing a link between total serum cholesterol levels and CHD but later more sophisticated studies allowed focus on the different types of lipoprotein and their effect on CHD. For example, the PROCAM study from Germany again highlights the dangerous association of low HDL, high triglyceride and moderately raised LDL (p. 119).

The Cholesterol Papers

The association between serum cholesterol and CHD has recently been examined again in an influential overview by Law *et al.* (1994) who published three papers addressing three major questions:

- the strength of the relationship between serum cholesterol and CHD;
- the extent and time course of CHD reduction with a given degree of cholesterol reduction;
- the possible adverse effects of cholesterol lowering (Chapter 3).

In the first paper, the authors used data from 21 515 males aged 35–64 years attending the British United Provident Association (BUPA) centre in London between 1975 and 1982. In the follow-up to 1991, there were 538 deaths. Two statistical corrections were applied to the results to prevent underestimation of the association between serum cholesterol and CHD:

1. *Regression Dilution Bias*
   This factor corrects for the natural variation of serum cholesterol within an individual over time and also for variation in laboratory measurement. Single measurement for a cohort study might place an individual in a false risk quintile and this adds bias.
2. *Surrogate Dilution Effect*
   Cohort studies tend to measure total serum cholesterol, 1 mmol/l in total cholesterol being equivalent to 0.67 mmol/l of LDL cholesterol. Intervention studies show that a 1 mmol/l drop in total cholesterol is equivalent to a 1 mmol/l drop in LDL because it is LDL that is lowered by diet and drugs. It follows that extrapolations of the effect of lower cholesterol from cohort trials will underestimate the associated rate of CHD.

The paper analysed the BUPA data to produce a figure for reduction in CHD associated with a reduction of 0.6 mmol/l total cholesterol. This figure was chosen because it was roughly 10% of the UK average and the sort of improvement that could be brought about by life style and dietary change.

For every 0.6 mmol/l reduction in total cholesterol, there were reductions in CHD of 17%, 24% when corrected for RDB and 27% when corrected for SDE. Moreover, all-cause mortality after correction was also reduced by 10%, i.e. a 10% reduction in cholesterol led to a 10% reduction in total mortality.

The second paper, using data from the 10 largest cohort studies (including MRFIT, BRHS, BUPA and Whitehall) and three international studies (including Seven Countries, and Ni Hon San), extended the statistical corrections to a cumulative database of nearly half a million men. This time, for every 0.6 mmol/l reduction in total cholesterol. CHD in the cohort studies was reduced by 54% at 40 years, 39% at 50 years, 27% at 60 years, 20% at 70 years and 19% at 80 years, and in the international studies by 38% at 55–64 years.

Although the reduction of cholesterol is weaker with increasing age, the absolute effects are greater. It is estimated that a 54% reduction in CHD in males aged 40 would save 400 deaths/year in the UK whereas a reduction of 19% at 80 would save 20 000.

If a 30% drop in cholesterol (1.8 mmol/l) such as observed in the 4S Study is used as the baseline cholesterol reduction, the postponement of CHD death is predicted to average 9 years for a 60-year-old man.

The other findings of Law's papers are discussed in Chapter 3 (p.52).

Normal cholesterol levels

We have seen that serum cholesterol is distributed almost normally through a population and that the mean value differs with age and sex. We have also seen that the mean value is raised in countries with high rates of CHD. Most CHD events occur near to the mean due to the influence of other risk factors. The mean value of serum cholesterol for a population should not be construed as normal.

Laboratories tend to express results in terms of standard deviations from the mean, some suggesting a 'normal range' for cholesterol of 5.2 mmol/l to 7.8 mmol/l. Although levels of less than 5.2 mmol/l can be considered as 'normal' in most cases even at these levels some CHD events occur and it should be remembered that the relationship between serum cholesterol and CHD is continuous and graded.

CHOLESTEROL LEVELS IN GENERAL PRACTICE

Table 2.10 shows the percentage of the UK population with blood levels above certain accepted cholesterol thresholds. Translated to a five-partner practice of 10 000 patients, there would be about 3000 patients in the 25–59 age group. Approximately 2000 patients would have raised cholesterol levels of which at least 750 would be at significant risk (150 per partner). The burden of this work is beyond the resource of secondary care and, like hypertension, cholesterol management must become a primary care discipline.

Table 2.10
Percentage of UK population with blood levels above accepted cholesterol thresholds

Threshold (mmol/l)	Mann 1988	OPCS 1986–1987	MONICA (Scotland) 1984–1986
<5.2	34	34	25
5.2–6.5	41	39	39
6.5–7.8	21	20	25
>7.8	4	7	11

Populations, individuals, governments and the food industry

The underlying premise of the population strategy (see p.86) is that it seeks to change features of behaviour or the environment that are responsible for the overall rate of CHD. In essence this means informing and motivating the population to modify dietary, smoking and exercise habits. Central government should stimulate public education through health professionals, educationalists and the media. Local government can influence schools, industry, shops, restaurants and the provision of exercise facilities. Sadly, changes are more often dictated by public demand, although there is evidence to suggest that a coordinated approach can be effective (e.g. the Minnesota Heart Health Project and the North Karelia project in Finland).

If, for example, British Dietary Reference Values were to be adopted in the UK, mean serum cholesterol levels in 25–60 year olds would be expected to be reduced by approximately 12% from about 6.0 to 5.2 mmol/l (Figure 2.15). Compliance with the more restrictive WHO dietary recommendations would lead to a greater fall (of 17%) and a major distribution shift in the prevalence of hypercholesterolaemia. Moreover, as cholesterol-lowering diets tend also to be weight optimizing, the fall in numbers with obesity would also further shift the cholesterol curve.

The right of an individual 'to die as I choose' often baulks the best efforts of health professionals to induce life style change. Too often this is rooted in ignorance and ill informed traditional belief. The counters to this include not only information, education and motivation but also government-directed democratically developed social policy. Individual restrictions for the good of others already exist – for example, the use of seat belts, drink/driving regulations, restrictions in the sale of tobacco and alcohol, and advertising limitations. The effect of increasing tobacco taxation is linked to a decline in smoking but much more could be done to reduce the social acceptability of smoking.

The fact that food production in much of Europe is still linked to the nutritional priorities of the 1950s has led to massive agricultural surpluses, particularly surplus animal products and especially from the dairy industry (Table 2.11). This has led to the introduction of quotas and subsidies which have not only maintained production values but also flooded poorer countries (e.g. Eastern Europe) with excess cheap saturated fat.

Until recently, meat carcasses were appraised for quality on their 'shape', 'finish' and 'marbling', all reflective of increased fat content and luxury status. There is now increased demand for lower fat meats and this is most dramatically met in pig farming, where lean pork now contains less fat than chicken. Intensive feeding practices by poultry farmers have raised fat content compared with free-range varieties. Unfortunately dairy cows, whose breeding attracts subsidized payments, tend to produce a high fat meat. Similarly, castrated bulls produce a high fat meat unless treated with anabolic steroids. Excess fatty meat that cannot be sold direct is then incorporated into meat products, sausages, meat

Figure 2.15
Differences between
recommended and
current diet in the UK.
Source: Ball and Mann
(1994)

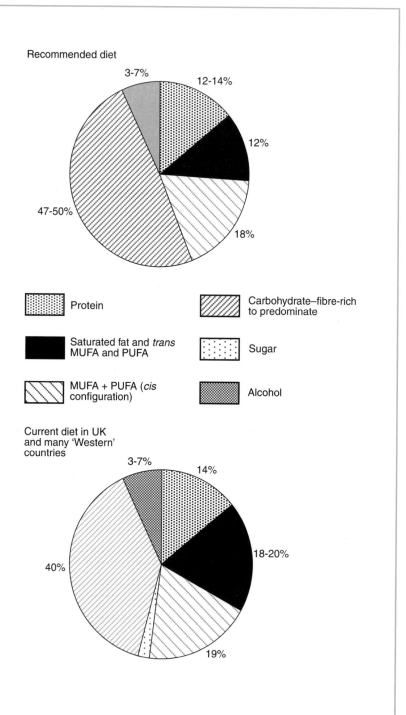

pies, salamis, etc. which, being cheaper, are more attractive to the economically deprived.

In the UK, 70% of products are now packaged or manufactured and are often high in hidden salt and sugar, providing an invisible intake for the consumer. Salt content is increased to allow for greater water content, thereby increasing bulk and ultimately profit.

To offset these hidden problems in nutrition, there is obviously a need for compulsory standardized food labelling, using language that is comprehensible to ordinary people. For example, bread is probably our chief source of salt currently with a content as high as 1.1 g sodium/100 g. Consumers might purchase lower-salt brands if they were aware that this amount comfortably exceeds the concentration in sea water (0.9 g sodium/100g).

In summary, the consumer is faced with a number of dilemmas when aiming to choose the components of a healthy diet (Figure 2.16).

There are clear roles for government:

1. To establish an independent food protection agency to protect the public from misleading information and institute better food labelling.
2. To review agricultural strategies.
3. To establish services to implement and publicize health recommendations, particularly nutrition education, smoking policies and the facilitation of exercise.

Fat source	Percentage of total fat consumption
Butter and margarines	16%
Meat	14%
Milk	9%
Vegetables (including chips and crisps)	11%
Cheese	6%
Meat products	10%
Cakes, biscuits, puddings	19%
Other fats (e.g. cooking oil, etc.)	15%

Table 2.11
Fat consumption in the UK (OPCS, 1990)

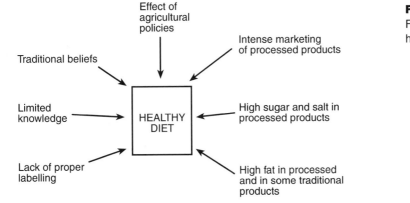

Figure 2.16
Factors affecting a healthy diet.

Lipid-lowering trials

3

Many trials of lipid lowering with various diet and drug therapies have been conducted during the last three decades but until 1994 no trial reported an unequivocal result. Over the years these trials have caused much controversy not only in the medical press but also in the lay press. The controversy arose because of the failure of the trials to demonstrate overall benefit.

In the majority of trials the primary end-point was a combination of non-fatal and fatal myocardial infarction. Most commentators accepted that these events were reduced, but the reduction in CHD deaths did not translate into an improvement in overall mortality because there was an apparent excess of non-CHD deaths. This led to the well-known statement, probably first made by the late Professor Mitchell (then Professor of Medicine at Nottingham University), that the only effect of reducing cholesterol is to change the diagnosis on the gravestone. Instead of dying of CHD, patients on cholesterol-lowering therapy would die of other causes, principally cancer and, of particular interest because it attracted so much attention in the lay press, suicide or violent deaths.

The fact that the early trials did not have the statistical power to determine effects on overall mortality did not seem to deter the principal protagonists of the 'let's attack the cholesterol story' brigade. The effect on patients was often – as might be expected – very distressing, as various startling headlines appeared in the lay press. This situation was compounded by the fact (still a problem with all the major weekly medical journals) that controversial information becomes available to the lay press prior to receipt of the relevant journal by its subscribers. This led to immense problems during the height of the so-called cholesterol controversy in trying to deal with calls from concerned patients.

This problem is well illustrated by an article in the *British Medical Journal* (*BMJ*) in 1992 entitled 'For debate: should there be a moratorium on the use of cholesterol-lowering drugs?' (Smith and Pekkanen, 1992). A particularly outrageous headline based on this article appeared in *The Guardian* (February 14, 1992): 'Murders Linked to Low Fat Drugs!' Imagine reading that headline if you were a patient on drug therapy. The *BMJ* report was even predicted in *The Sunday Times* the week before publication. Under the headline 'Health Call' it was reported that 'a moratorium on using cholesterol-lowering drugs is to be urged after evidence that they do not reduce – and may increase – death rates. A study in the *British Medical Journal* by researchers at the London School of Hygiene and Tropical Medicine confirms December's *Sunday Times* report that cutting cholesterol can be bad for you in certain circumstances.' In these circumstances it was difficult for physicians to reassure patients as the relevant *BMJ* issue had not by then reached its subscribers. When debate about important issues in medicine is conducted in this way it is often the headline message which is accepted by the profession as well as the patient.

The controversy arose because the cholesterol-lowering trials lacked the statistical power to provide a definitive analysis of overall mortality. In most trials there was no significant difference in non-CHD deaths (apart from the WHO collaborative trial of clofibrate which is discussed later) but there were, literally, one or two more deaths in the drug treatment group from cancer or suicide or violent death – the most likely explanation being a chance effect.

In an attempt to address these possible adverse effects it became fashionable to adopt the technique of meta-analysis which emerged in the 1980s. The potential advantages and disadvantages of this technique are shown in Table 3.1. The application of the technique (which, by combining the results of similar trials, increases the statistical power for testing a treatment benefit or adverse effect) led to widely different conclusions in regard to the cholesterol story. Meta-analyses particularly highlighted the possibility of increased suicide and violent death in relation to cholesterol lowering (Muldoon *et al.*, 1990; Smith and Pekkanen, 1992). This disturbing claim was reiterated so many times that it was accepted as fact and hypotheses were published to explain the phenomenon. This was irksome to those of us working in the subject because researchers from the Food and Drug Association (FDA) had undertaken a detailed review of such deaths in the two largest trials where there appeared to be an issue and published their findings in 1990 (Wysowski and Gross, 1990).

In the Lipid Research Clinics (LRC) primary prevention trial using the anion exchange resin, cholestyramine (Lipid Research Clinics Programme, 1984), four individuals in the treatment group committed suicide, compared with two taking placebo. Of the four cases (three by gunshot wounds to the head and one by hanging) there was a history in three of tranquillizer use or psychiatric symptoms at entry into the study. Furthermore three of the cases dropped out of the study. Only one suicide case showed good compliance with the study drug and had no previous history of psychiatric symptoms. In the study as a whole there were no differences in the

Advantages	Disadvantages
Increased patient numbers and therefore increased statistical power to detect treatment differences	Potential for bias from publication bias and choice of trials for inclusion/exclusion in the analysis
Identification of subgroups who do well (or badly)	Post hoc nature of the analysis
A robust test of whether the results can be generalized	'Similar' trials may have important differences, e.g. disease severity; therefore equivalent to combining apples, pears, etc.
Neutralization of extreme results (positive or negative) of individual trials	

Meta-analysis: a pooled analysis that employs formal statistical methods to combine outcome results from clinical trials of particular therapeutic interventions.

Table 3.1
Advantages and disadvantages of meta-analysis (Furberg and Furberg, 1994)

incidence of psychiatric symptoms or the use of antidepressants during the trial.

With regard to accidental deaths in the LRC study there were six in the drug-treated group compared with two on placebo. Alcohol was detected at autopsy in three cases and was a possible factor in two others; also, the nature of some of the accidents suggested intoxication (a head-on collision while using a mobile phone and a single-car accident). Two of the accidents were probably unavoidable – a car driver was hit by a trailer which had broken loose from an oncoming truck and a motor cyclist was struck from behind by a hit-and-run driver. Compliance with the study drug in three of the cases was poor and four had a history of either tranquillizer use or psychiatric symptoms prior to the trial. In the six cases the average cholesterol was 6.46 mmol/l.

The other trial that contributed to the suicide and violent death controversy was the Helsinki Heart Study (HHS) (Frick *et al.*, 1987) with the fibrate, gemfibrozil. In this study there were four suicides on gemfibrozil and two on placebo. Two cases in the treatment group were study drop-outs. Of the remainder, the mean cholesterol at the last study visit was 6.7 mmol/l. Based on population characteristics, 11 suicides should have been expected during the study and so the frequency of suicide observed was less than expected in both the drug and the placebo groups. There were four fatal accidents in the gemfibrozil group and four in the placebo group. Two of the accident cases were study drop-outs and alcohol was detected at post mortem. In the treatment group mean cholesterol at the last study visit was 7.2 mmol/l.

Remember the *Guardian* headline about murders? Indeed there were two murders – one in the LRC study and one in the Helsinki study – but the trial participants were victims, not perpetrators of the crime. It would be interesting to consider the biochemical and cellular mechanisms induced by taking a lipid-lowering drug that are likely to lead to an increased risk of being a murder victim.

The conclusion of the meticulous analysis of Wysowski and Gross (1990) for the FDA on suicide and violent death was that 'when drop-outs and known risk factors for the deaths such as alcohol intoxication and psychiatric histories are considered, little evidence remains to support the hypothesis that cholesterol-lowering drugs are causally associated with deaths due to homicides, suicides and accidents in these trials'.

When the cholesterol-lowering trials were analysed (and up to 1993 there were nearly 50 controlled clinical trials involving approximately 85 000 participants) widely different conclusions were frequently obtained, often when similar data were examined. For instance, Holme (1990) found a strong correlation across the various trials between reductions in cholesterol level and mortality and pointed to the trend for mortality reduction when cholesterol was reduced by over 9%. On the other hand, Ravnskov (1992) concluded that cholesterol lowering was unlikely to lower CHD, let alone overall mortality.

Fortunately there have been attempts to put the record straight with regard to the cholesterol trials. For those interested in pursuing the history of meta-analysis in this area, the Further Reading section provides a source of excellent analyses.

In an important contribution that comprised the third of the Cholesterol Papers (Chapter 2) published in the *BMJ*, Law *et al.*, (1994c) examined the possible hazards of reducing serum cholesterol. Previous meta-analyses of selected cholesterol lowering trials showed an apparent excess of non-CHD deaths, particularly suicides and violent death and possibly cancer. These small excesses, likely to be the play of chance, were nevertheless linked to epidemiological studies that demonstrated an upturn in overall mortality in the lowest part of the cholesterol distribution.

Law and colleagues analysed data from the ten largest cohort studies, two international studies and 28 randomized trials of cholesterol lowering – the mean outcome measure being excess cause-specific mortality with low or lowered cholesterol concentration. Non-CHD deaths were divided into other circulatory diseases, cancer, accidents and suicides, and other causes.

The question whether low cholesterol concentration predisposes to illness or whether low cholesterol is secondary to illness was addressed in an interesting way. The authors divided the available cohorts into those that recruited from employed populations and those that recruited from populations as a whole. The reasonable assumption is that those individuals in employment are on the whole likely to be healthier. No excess mortality was found associated with low cholesterol in cohorts of employed people. On the other hand there was a significant excess mortality in the community cohorts. Law and colleagues interpreted these findings as evidence that preceding illness was likely to be the explanation for the low cholesterol/non-CHD death association seen in the community cohorts. The authors did find an excess of non-CHD deaths when they analysed the controlled trials but pointed to the difficulties of reaching meaningful conclusions, because of the small number of deaths in the studies, their relatively short duration and the fact that low cholesterol levels were not achieved.

In order further to assess possible hazards due to low cholesterol they examined data from cohorts and international comparisons. They found no overall excess of cancer deaths in the randomized trials. This finding, together with observations from prospective studies showing that a low cholesterol/cancer association present at baseline and in the early years of follow-up disappeared with continued follow-up, suggests that the association is due to the well described phenomenon that plasma cholesterol is reduced by cancers. The metabolic basis for this has been studied and increased LDL plasma clearance has been described in patients with malignancy, presumably to provide membrane cholesterol for the proliferating cells.

A difference between the employed and community cohorts was found for accidents and suicides, with a significant excess in the community cohorts in those with the lowest cholesterols (relative risk 1.48). Such an association was not found in the cohorts of employed people and in the international comparisons. The authors' conclusion was that the association could be explained by the plasma cholesterol reduction associated with the anorexia and weight loss of depression. As with the cancer association, the relationship of low cholesterol with suicide disappears after five years of follow-up. Importantly, no excess of accidents and suicides was seen overall in the randomized trials.

With regard to circulatory disorders other than CHD, Law and colleagues did conclude that the low cholesterol/haemorrhagic stroke association observed in cohort studies was likely to be causal in the presence of fairly high blood pressure. However the increased mortality from haemorrhagic stroke is small when compared with the lower CHD mortality. For instance, in the large MRFIT database, mortality from haemorrhagic stroke in men with the lowest cholesterol concentration ($<$ 4.14 mmol/1) was 0.3 per 10 000 man years higher when compared with that in the next lowest concentration (4.14–15 mmol/l). However, CHD mortality was 3.3 per 10 000 man years lower. Despite this conclusion, stroke overall in the three subsequent large statin trials (4S, WOSCOPS and CARE) was reduced.

Other-cause mortality (not cancer, accidents and suicides, and non-CHD circulatory disorders) was also investigated. There was a significant excess in the community studies (1.62) but again no excess was observed in the employed cohorts. Excess mortality was mainly related to chronic respiratory disorders and liver and bowel diseases. The authors concluded that the observed association was likely to be explained by the cholesterol-lowering effect of chronic disease. No excess of other-cause mortality was observed in the randomized trials or international comparisons.

There is no doubt that the monumental piece of work by Law and colleagues summarized above did much to reassure physicians about the safety of cholesterol lowering. Their final conclusion merits quoting in full (Law *et al.*, 1994c):

> The evidence is clear: the need is not to repeat research which has already been performed but to disseminate results, their interpretation and the conclusions so that preventive action can be taken to confer the substantial health benefit of lowering average serum cholesterol concentrations in Western populations.

As well as assessing the potential hazards of low cholesterol and lowering cholesterol, Law and colleagues (1994) provided an overview of cholesterol-lowering trials available up to 1994. The analysis is shown in Table 3.2. It concerned 28 randomized trials involving 46 254 men with 4241 reported CHD events. The trials chosen were randomized and controlled; they involved lipid lowering with diet and drugs and one trial of surgical intervention by partial ileal bypass. All the trials documented at least one

Table 3.2
Meta-analysis of cholesterol-lowering trials (Law *et al.*, 1994): percentage reduction of ischaemic heart disease events in men associated with a 0.6 mmol/l reduction in cholesterol (approximately 10%) by duration of trials

Trials	Time since entry to trial		
	$<$ 2 years	2.1–5 years	5.1–12 years
	Percentage reduction in IHD events		
All drug trials	10	21	22
All dietary trials	9	14	37
Trials of men without known ischaemic heart disease	11	25	24
Trials of men with ischaemic heart disease	6	20	24
All trials (95% confidence)	7 (0–14)	22 (15–28)	25 (15–35)

death and were associated with a cholesterol reduction of at least 1%. Trials that used what transpired to be noxious agents (oestrogen in men, and *d*-thyroxine) and that intervened on multiple risk factors were omitted.

The trials adopted similar diagnostic criteria for non-fatal myocardial infarction and CHD death and the assessment of these events was blinded as to treatment. All trials were analysed by intention to treat – that is, on the basis of the allocated treatment whether or not the treatment was actually taken. This is important to avoid bias.

As can be seen, the trials were analysed according to the nature of the intervention (diet or drug), the study population (with and without existing symptomatic coronary heart disease) and the duration of the trials. The results of meta-analysis were expressed as CHD risk reduction associated with a reduction of serum cholesterol concentration of 0.6 mmol/l. This figure was chosen because it represents approximately 10% of the average cholesterol concentrations seen in Western countries.

As might be expected, the observed benefit of cholesterol lowering increased with increasing duration of cholesterol reduction and overall there was a highly significant reduction in non-fatal (21%; $P < 0.001$) events and also in CHD death (10%; $P = 0.004$) for a 0.6 mmol/l cholesterol reduction. Most trials excluded women but the small amount of data available from three of the trials that did include women showed significant reduction in CHD events of similar magnitude to that for men (Law *et al.*, 1994b).

Primary prevention trials

When these trials are critically evaluated, there is no doubt that they illustrate a learning curve with regard to the design, conduct, statistical analysis and reporting of clinical trials. Defects in clinical trial technology in the past have contributed to the cholesterol controversy.

It is important for the individual physician to be in a position to evaluate published trials. This skill was not taught when the authors were at medical school. Fortunately this particular inadequacy has since been remedied and considerable attention is now paid to the design and evaluation of clinical trials in undergraduate clinical pharmacology courses. Nevertheless it is worth a little general revision.

The writings of the Furbergs (Bengt and Curt) on the subject of clinical trials are thoroughly recommended – in particular a book entitled *All That Glitters is not Gold: What clinicians need to know about clinical trials* (published by Dr Potata, Winston-Salem, USA, 1994). A distillation of what the Furbergs refer to as the 'road map for reading trial results' is shown in Table 3.3.

With regard to the cholesterol-lowering trials the principal defects over the years have been:

- lack of statistical power to test effects on CHD death or overall mortality;
- lack of effective intervention, leading to small differences in cholesterol between treated and placebo groups;
- small numbers of observed CHD events and death due to exclusion of high-risk patients.

In the overview of the cholesterol-lowering trials by Law *et al.* (1994b) it is clear that the early primary prevention trials do demonstrate a significant reduction in CHD events. However, no reduction – or even a slight excess – of non-CHD events was observed. The increase in non-CHD deaths was not due to any particular cause. This fits with the hazards analysis by the same authors, which examined not only the trials but also international comparisons and cohort studies. The significant overall increase in non-

Table 3.3
'Road map' for evaluating clinical trial reports according to the Furbergs (1994)

> ► Is the scientific question clearly stated and are the results important to my patients and clinical practice?
> ► What were the selection criteria and are they applicable to my patients?
> ► Were the dosing and treatment periods adequate?
> ► Was the trial of sufficient size to allow the detection of moderate but clinically meaningful differences?
> ► Were the placebo and treated groups well matched at baseline and were data on concomitant other therapies and diseases described?
> ► To minimize potential bias:
>   – Was treatment allocation randomized and double-blind?
>   – Was the assessment of treatment outcomes blinded to treatment groups?
> ► Were all randomized patients accounted for in the final analysis?
> ► Are the negative effects of the treatment thoroughly documented?
> ► Are the results consistent with other similar, well conducted studies?
> ► Do the benefits outweigh the risks and associated costs?
> ► Are the authors sufficiently independent of any potential conflicts of interest that could cast doubt on the objectivity of the trial?

CHD deaths in the early trials appeared for the most part to be due to the first fibrate drug, clofibrate, and the hormone trials (oestrogen and *d*-thyroxine), (Law *et al.*, 1994c).

It was the WHO clofibrate trial that was mainly responsible for the excess non-CHD deaths in the drug trials (Committee of Principal Investigators, 1978). In this trial the excess mortality was attributed to cancer and hepatobiliary disease. It is known that clofibrate increases the lithogenicity of bile and therefore gallstone formation. For this reason the drug is now largely redundant. Several of the deaths in the WHO trial were indeed associated with gall-bladder surgery. This trial will be described in detail later.

Some of the major primary prevention trials using diet and drug therapy will be discussed in detail here to provide a flavour of the trials and to provide the background for the recent landmark West of Scotland Primary Prevention trial – the first such study to employ one of the statin drugs.

OSLO STUDY

The Oslo study (Table 3.4a) is a particularly attractive trial in the sense that it took as its study population a group of men considered to be at high CHD risk because of hypercholesterolaemia and intervened with dietary and anti-smoking advice – therapeutic options that are still first line for most physicians (Hjermann *et al.*, 1981). More than 16 000 men (aged 40–49 years) were screened for possible inclusion in this five-year randomized trial and 1232 asymptomatic men were selected with total serum cholesterol concentrations of 7.5–9.8 mmol/l. Eighty per cent were smokers.

The 604 men randomly allocated to the treatment arm of the study were prescribed a cholesterol-lowering diet and were given anti-smoking advice. Over the course of the study there was an approximately 13% reduction in serum cholesterol and a 45% reduction in tobacco consumption. At the end of the study 25% of men had stopped cigarette smoking compared with 17% in the non-intervention group.

Over the five-year course of the study there was a 47% reduction in the combined end-point of fatal and non-fatal myocardial infarction and sudden death in the intervention group compared with the control group ($P = 0.028$). Two-thirds of this benefit was attributed to cholesterol reduction. Follow-up of the study participants at 42 months after the end of the trial showed a 40% reduction in overall mortality which was marginally significant.

The results of the Oslo study confirmed those of earlier dietary intervention trials, such as the Los Angeles Veterans Study (Dayton *et al.*, 1969) (Table 3.4b) and the Finnish Mental Hospitals study (Turpeinen, 1979)

(a) Oslo Primary Prevention Trial (Hjermann *et al*., 1981)

Study participants:
men aged 40–49 years
(*n* = 1232) with
hypercholesterolaemia
(≥ 7.5 mmol/l); 80% were
smokers

Five-year randomized trial of
cholesterol-lowering diet and
anti-smoking advice

In the intervention group serum
cholesterol was reduced by 13%
and tobacco consumption fell by
65%. In the intervention group
25% quit cigarette smoking,
compared with 17% in the
control group

End-point effects (number of
episodes):

	Control (*n* = 628)	(*n* = 604)
Coronary heart disease	36	19*
All cardio-vascular disease	39	22*
Total cardio-vascular death	15	8
Sudden death	11	3*
Total deaths	24	16

(b) Los Angeles Veterans Study (Dayton *et al*., 1969)

Study participants:
men, mean age ~ 65
years, (*n* = 846) resident
in a Veterans
Administration Hospital

Eight-year randomized
double-blind study of usual
diet vs. modified fat diet
(PS ratio 2.0)

Mean reduction in total
serum cholesterol 13% on
experimental diet

Results (experimental vs.
usual diet, *P*< 0.05):
CHD deaths, 48 vs. 70
Atherosclerotic events, 66
vs. 96
Benefits greatest in younger
men and those with higher
cholesterol levels
Increase in non-
cardiovascular deaths
This type of diet not now
used

(c) Finnish Mental Hospitals Study (Turpeinen, 1979)

Study participants:
inpatients of two mental
hospitals in Helsinki

Cross-over study of
cholesterol-lowering,
modified fat diet vs. usual
diet. One group received
experimental diet for six
years and the other the
usual diet and then
changed over

CHD deaths (experimental
vs. usual diet):
3.0 vs. 6.1 per 1000 man
years (NS)
CHD disease plus major
ECG changes
4.2 vs. 12.7 per 1000
man years (*P* <0.001)

Confounding factors:
patients were receiving a
variety of psychotropic
drugs; patients discharged
from hospital were lost to
the trial; patients admitted
during the trial were
enrolled
Applicability to 'free living'
people
No excess of non-
cardiovascular deaths

Table 3.4
Primary prevention trials; *P* < 0.05

(Table 3.4c) which pointed to the potential benefit of the lipid-lowering diet. The Oslo study had the great advantage of a free-living population, as opposed to institutionalized participants in the other two studies.

WHO COOPERATIVE TRIAL OF CLOFIBRATE

This trial was the first major primary prevention trial of drug therapy and was initiated in the mid 1960s in three major European cities – Budapest, Edinburgh and Prague, (Committee of Principal Investigators, 1978). About 30 000 men (aged 30–59 years) were screened for possible inclusion in the trial. Approximately 10 000 men whose cholesterol fell in the upper third of the distribution were randomly allocated to double-blind treatment with either clofibrate, 1.6 g/day ($n = 5331$), or placebo capsules containing olive oil ($n = 5296$).

Over the course of the study (5.3 years) clofibrate therapy was associated with a net cholesterol reduction of 8% (the baseline cholesterol was $\simeq 6.4$ mmol/l) and this was associated with an overall reduction in CHD events (167 events on clofibrate vs. 207 on placebo), mainly attributable to a 25% reduction in non-fatal events. There was no significant reduction in fatal events, though this would be difficult to show as the incidence of fatal infarction was very low at 0.7%.

The favourable effect of clofibrate on CHD events was overshadowed by an increase in total deaths in the clofibrate-treated group (162 on clofibrate vs. 127 on placebo). This was due to an increase in non-CHD deaths (94 vs. 65) with no difference in CHD deaths (68 vs. 62). It is important to note that no particular cause of death was found to be in excess. However, the causes of death relating to 'liver, gall-bladder and intestines' and the increased frequency of cholecystectomy are likely to relate to the biliary lithogenic effect of clofibrate.

Withdrawals from the clofibrate group during the trial were more frequent than those from the placebo group (346 vs. 327). Gallstone operations, weight gain, indigestion, diarrhoea, diabetes and impotence were significantly more frequent in the clofibrate group.

The design of the WHO trial has been much criticized, particularly with regard to the analysis of the mortality data. The study design did not allow for in-trial results to be presented on an intention-to-treat analysis. Furthermore, the out-of-trial mortality follow-up data were incomplete. Taking this into account, there is no doubt that the most reliable data from the study related to the numbers of non-fatal myocardial infarction as participants were withdrawn from the trial after these events.

Recently the principal investigators of the WHO Cooperative study have published their intention to treat analysis of the results (Heady *et al.*, 1992).

This analysis still showed an excess of non-cardiac deaths without any significant excess of particular causes of death.

In relation to the excess non-CHD deaths in this study it is worth considering the other large clofibrate trial which formed one treatment arm of the Coronary Drug Project (CDP) secondary prevention trial (Coronary Drug Project Research Group, 1975). In the clofibrate group ($n = 1103$ men) there was no significant increase in non-CHD mortality during six years of study.

LIPID RESEARCH CLINICS (LRC) CORONARY PRIMARY PREVENTION TRIAL

This large, well-designed trial was reported in 1984 (Lipid Research Clinics Programme, 1984) and its results prompted guidelines to be drawn up in the United States for the treatment of hypercholesterolaemia for the prevention of CHD.

The study population consisted of asymptomatic men aged 35–59 years with a cholesterol level greater than the 95th centile for the US population, approximately 6.8 mmol/l. The average baseline concentration was 7.5 mmol/l and individuals with triglyceride concentrations greater than 3.4 mmol/l were excluded.

3806 men were recruited and randomly allocated to the anion exchange resin cholestyramine (24 g/day; $n = 1906$) or placebo ($n = 1900$). In addition to the study medication all participants received lipid-lowering dietary advice, which produced a mean cholesterol reduction of 4%.

Over the study period (mean follow up 7.4 years) the net fall in serum cholesterol in the cholestyramine group compared with placebo was 9% and for LDL cholesterol 13% (Table 3.5). The power of the study was based on a 25% reduction in serum cholesterol in the treated group but was not achieved because of compliance problems with the resin, which is difficult to take. Therefore the power of the study was reduced. Nevertheless, there was a significant reduction in the primary end-point of the study (definite CHD event – fatal or non-fatal), with 155 events in the cholestyramine group vs. 187 events in the placebo group ($P < 0.05$).

The principal finding is supported by other data from the study which shows a pleasing consistency in relation to cholesterol lowering with cholestyramine. For instance, other secondary CHD end-points showed similar reductions (Table 3.5) Furthermore, because of the variation in compliance already mentioned it was possible to examine the relationship between the degree of LDL lowering and CHD events (Table 3.6). The one-third of individuals with LDL cholesterol reductions of more than 25% showed a 64% reduction in myocardial infarction.

End-point	Placebo (n = 1900)		Cholestyramine (n = 1906)		Risk reduction (%)
	No.	%	No.	%	
(a) Primary end-points					
Definite CHD death and/or definite non-fatal infarction	187*	9.8	155*	8.1	19
Definite or suspect CHD death or non-fatal infarction	256*	13.5	222*	11.6	15
All-cause mortality	71	3.7	68	3.6	7
(b) Secondary end-points					
CHD:					
Positive exercise test	345	19.8*	260	14.9*	25*
Angina	287	15.1*	235	12.4*	20*
Coronary bypass surgery	112	5.9	93	4.9	21*
Congestive heart failure	11	0.6	8	0.4	28
Intraoperative myocardial infarction	7	0.4	5	0.3	29
Resuscitated coronary collapse	5	0.3	3	0.2	40
Cerebrovascular Disease:					
Definite or suspect transient ischaemia attack	22	1.2	18	0.9	18
Definite or suspect atherothrombotic brain infarction	14	0.7	17	0.9	+21
Peripheral Vascular Disease:					
Intermittent claudication	84	4.4*	72	3.8*	15

* Statistically significant.
Study participants: men aged 35–59 years with primary hypercholesterolaemia; 7.4-year randomized controlled trial of cholestyramine, 24 g/day (n = 1906) vs. placebo (n = 1900), both groups receiving cholesterol-lowering diet. In treated group, net reduction of serum cholesterol = 9% and of LDL cholesterol = 13%.

Table 3.5
Primary and secondary end-points of Lipid Research Clinics (LRC) Coronary Primary Prevention Study (Lipid Research Clinics Programme, 1984).

Table 3.6

Compliance with cholestyramine and reduction of serum cholesterol: relationship to CHD risk[a]

Packet count	No.	Total cholesterol & reduction	CHD events % reduction
0–2	439	4.4	10.9
2–5	496	11.5	26.1
5–6	965	19.0	39.3

[a] Source: Lipid Research Clinics Program, 1984, *J. Am. Med. Assoc.*, **251**, 351

There was no difference in overall mortality (68 deaths in the cholestyramine group vs. 71 deaths in the placebo group). There was no difference in cancer deaths. As discussed elsewhere, some commentators made much of the small, non-significant excess of deaths from accidents and violence (11 on cholestyramine vs. 4 on placebo).

Adverse effects encountered during the study were predictably (given the drug used) related to the gastrointestinal tract. In the first year gastrointestinal symptoms were reported in 64% of participants on cholestyramine compared with 43% on placebo.

HELSINKI HEART STUDY (HHS)

This major primary prevention trial (Frick *et al.*, 1987) differs from the LRC trial in several respects. Firstly the trial drug used, gemfibrozil, is a second generation fibrate and secondly the lipid entry criteria (non-HDL cholesterol ≥ 5.2 mmol/l) led to inclusion of individuals with lipoprotein phenotypes (28% IIb; 9% IV) (see Table 5.1) other than isolated hypercholesterolaemia (63% IIa). Baseline lipid concentrations were: total cholesterol 6.9 mmol/l, total triglyceride 2.0 mmol/l and HDL cholesterol 1.2 mmol/l.

All participants (men aged 40–55 years) were advised on a lipid-lowering diet and 2051 men were randomly allocated to gemfibrozil (1.2 g/day) and 2031 to placebo.

The lipid changes achieved in the study are shown in Table 3.7. Not surprisingly these changes were in part dependent on the lipoprotein phenotype – apart from the increase in HDL cholesterol, which was roughly equivalent.

After a mean five year follow-up period there was a significant 35% reduction in the primary study end point of combined non-fatal and fatal myocardial infarction (56 events on gemfibrozil v.s 84 on placebo). As in the LRC study there was no difference in overall mortality (45 deaths on gemfibrozil vs. 42 deaths on placebo). However, as discussed elsewhere, the study did not have the statistical power to determine effects on mortality. Cancer deaths were identical (11 vs. 11) and there was a non-significant excess of deaths from accidents and violence in the gemfibrozil group (5 vs. 1).

Adverse effects in the gemfibrozil group during the study period were mainly related to the gastrointestinal tract (11% vs. 7%). Of particular interest, in view of the findings of the WHO clofibrate study, was the incidence of gall-bladder surgery. There were 18 operations in the gemfibrozil group compared with 12 in the placebo group, which did not reach statistical significance.

In multivariate regression analysis the benefit observed in the HHS was related to both the reduction in LDL cholesterol and the increase in HDL cholesterol. In an interesting post hoc analysis it was found that much of the benefit of gemfibrozil occurred in individuals with cholesterol/HDL cholesterol ratios greater than 5 who were also hypertriglyceridaemic. This is discussed on p. 120.

Table 3.7
Helsinki Heart Study (Frick *et al.*, 1987)

Study participants:
  men aged 40–55 years ($n = 4082$)
  with non-HDL cholesterol ≥ 5.2 mmol/l;
  63% were Type II_a, 28% Type II_b and 9% Type IV

Five-year randomized trial of gemfibrozil (1200 mg/day) vs. placebo

Lipid and lipoprotein changes in the gemfibrozil-treated group ($n = 2051$):

Cholesterol	10% net reduction
LDL cholesterol	11% net reduction
Triglyceride	35% net reduction
HDL cholesterol	11% net increase

Major end-point: a combination of fatal and non-fatal myocardial infarction – 54 treated vs. 84 placebo ($P < 0.02$)

No difference in overall mortality:
  45 deaths on gemfibrozil
  42 deaths on placebo

WEST OF SCOTLAND CORONARY PREVENTION STUDY (WOSCOPS)

This landmark study (Shepherd *et al.*, 1995) largely overcame the design defects in earlier primary prevention trials such that when all the information is available it will provide invaluable assistance in assessing CHD risk in middle-aged men, allowing the targeting of drug treatment to those at higher risk.

The design of WOSCOPS (West of Scotland Coronary Prevention Study Group, 1992) built on the information available from the LRC and HHS studies. It was designed to have the statistical power to address the question of cholesterol lowering and the prevention of coronary events (combined incidence of non-fatal myocardial infarction and death from CHD). In order to achieve this it was necessary to study a population with a higher event rate and to increase the sample size. In addition, with the advent of the statin class of drugs it was possible to use a more powerful and better tolerated drug.

Approximately 160 000 men were invited to attend cholesterol screening sessions in general practices in the West of Scotland district for possible inclusion in the trial and 81 161 attended. Of these, those whose non-fasting plasma cholesterol (using the Reflotron bench-top analyser) was greater than 6.5 mmol/l were given lipid-lowering dietary advice and asked to reattend in four weeks. At the second visit 20 914 men had a fasting lipid profile. At this occasion, if LDL cholesterol was at least 4.0 mmol/l and there were no exclusion criteria, individuals were recalled after a further four weeks of diet. At the third visit, which involved 13 654 men, a further lipoprotein profile was performed together with an electrocardiogram. At the fourth visit, randomization to trial drug (pravastatin, 40 mg daily) or placebo was performed if:

● fasting LDL cholesterol was at least 4.0 mmol/l, with one value of at least 4.5 mmol/l and one value below 6.0 mmol/l;
● there were no serious ECG abnormalities;
● there was no history of myocardial infarction.

The 6595 study participants were seen at three monthly intervals during the study, with a fasting lipid profile every six months and a physical examination every year. The mean study period was 4.9 years, providing 32 216 subject years of follow-up.

The effects of pravastatin on LDL cholesterol achieved during the study are shown in Figure 3.1 both on an intention-to-treat and actual treatment basis.

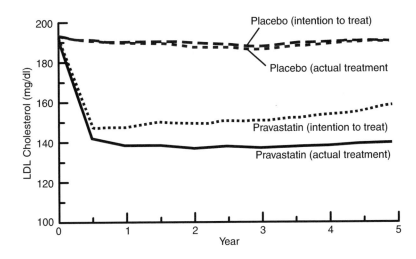

Figure 3.1
Effects of pravastatin therapy on plasma LDL cholesterol concentrations in the West of Scotland Coronary Prevention Study (to convert values for cholesterol to mmol/l, multiply by 0.026). Source: Shepherd *et al.* (1995).

The primary end-point of the study – death from CHD and definite non-fatal myocardial infarction – showed a 31% reduction (95% confidence intervals, 17–43%; $P < 0.001$) in the pravastatin group as compared with placebo. This result and effects on other secondary end-points are shown in Table 3.8. It can be seen that there was a significant reduction in CHD deaths and importantly this was not accompanied by an increase in non-cardiovascular deaths in the pravastatin group (56 vs. 62) such that overall mortality was also reduced. There were 116 individuals with cancer (fatal and non-fatal) in the pravastatin compared with 106 in the placebo group.

Pravastatin therapy was well-tolerated with little difference from the placebo group for myalgia or muscle pains. Four subjects (three pravastatin, one placebo) had asymptomatic episodes of high creatine phosphokinase levels (≥ 10 times normal). There were no cases of rhabdomyolysis and no significant differences in liver function tests between the pravastatin and placebo groups.

It is of interest that the same percentage benefits of pravastatin were seen whether or not LDL cholesterol or HDL cholesterol or triglyceride was above or below the median for the group. Furthermore, similar benefits were seen in smokers vs. non-smokers; those aged less than 55 years compared with those older than 55 years; and those with multiple risk factors vs. those without other risk factors.

This landmark trial has answered important questions on the benefit of lowering cholesterol in the prevention of CHD. This can be done safely with pravastatin and what is now needed is to identify a risk score for

Table 3.8
West of Scotland Coronary Prevention Study – results (Shepherd *et al.*, 1995)

Events and causes	Placebo (n = 3293)	Pravastatin (n = 3302)	P	Risk reduction % (95% CI)
Definite coronary events				
Non-fatal MI or CHD death	248	174	<0.001	31 (17–43)
Non-fatal MI	204	143	<0.001	31 (15–45)
CHD death	52	38	0.13	28 (–10–52)
Other events				
Coronary angiography	128	90	0.007	31 (10–47)
PTCA or CABG	80	51	0.009	37 (11–56)
Fatal or non-fatal stroke	51	46	0.57	11 (–33–40)
Incident cancer	106	116	0.55	–8 (–41–17)
Death from other causes				
Other cardiovascular causes, including stroke	12	9	–	–
Suicide	1	2	–	–
Trauma	5	3	–	–
Cancer	49	44	0.56	11 (–33–41)
All other causes	7	7	–	–
Deaths from all cardiovascular causes	73	50	0.033	32 (3–53)
Deaths from non-cardiovascular causes	62	56	0.54	11 (–28–38)
Deaths from any cause	135	106	0.051	22 (0–40)

patients based on the WOSCOPS data which will identify those at higher risk, so that therapy can be targeted on a cost-effective basis.

Secondary prevention trials

There is now overwhelming clinical trial evidence to justify aggressive lipid lowering in individuals with established CHD. Unfortunately, as the results of recent audits confirm, much still needs to be done to ensure that all patients have the opportunity to benefit clinically from current knowledge.

In this section an overview of the evidence linking cholesterol to outcome in those with manifest disease will be provided. The exciting findings of the angiographic and clinical events trials that have 'closed the loop' and demonstrated unequivocal benefits will be described.

Perhaps the early indication from trials such as the Coronary Drug Project (CDP) that the degree of myocardial infarction is the major determinant of outcome post infarction led to an impression that other factors, including cholesterol, were of little prognostic importance. There is no doubt of the importance of myocardial damage, particularly in the short term, but many studies in different populations have demonstrated that cholesterol is an important independent determinant of outcome in the long term.

Data from the Lipid Research Clinics Follow-up Study (LRC) (Pekkanen *et al.*, 1990) are shown in Figure 3.2. Increasing LDL cholesterol concentrations and decreasing HDL cholesterol concentrations are associated with risk of coronary death over 10 years of observation in men aged 40–69 years, both with and without clinical CHD. However, the observed

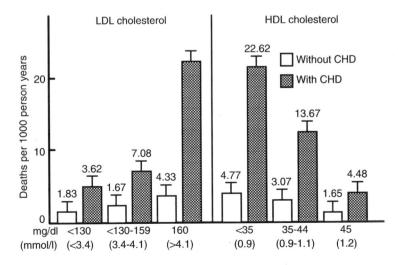

Figure 3.2
Lipid Research Clinics Follow-up Study. Relative risk of CHD death (age adjusted) in men (40–69 years) in relation to LDL and HDL cholesterol. Source: Pekkanen *et al.* (1990).

relationships are stronger in CHD patients. For instance, LDL cholesterol concentrations greater than 4.1 mmol/l are associated with a six-fold increased risk compared with concentrations of less than 3.4 mmol/l in patients with CHD. Similar findings have been reported from the Framingham study (Wong *et al.*, 1991), where information is also available on women. Cholesterol levels greater than 7 mmol/l were associated with a nine-fold increased CHD risk in women and a three-fold increased risk in men compared with levels of less than 5 mmol/l. In addition, all-cause mortality doubled with high cholesterol concentrations.

The potential for benefit of cholesterol reduction from observation studies such as the LRC and CDP is clear, as discussed by Rossouw *et al.* (1990) in an important overview in the *New England Journal of Medicine*. This article also provided a meta-analysis of lipid-lowering secondary prevention trials available up to that date. Using data from the LRC study it was calculated that if all the benefits could be obtained by reducing cholesterol from above 6.2 mmol/l (10-year CHD death risk, 170 per 1000) to below 5.2 mmol/l (16 per 1000) the potential saving of CHD death would be 154 per 1000. Obviously this presupposes that cholesterol lowering with diet or hypolipidaemic drugs, or both, would indeed deliver such a benefit. This can only be determined from controlled clinical trials.

EARLY TRIALS

Early secondary prevention trials suffered from many of the deficiencies discussed at the beginning of this section. Rossouw and colleagues set various criteria for inclusion of trials in their meta-analysis: at least 100 subjects in each treatment arm; a duration of at least three years; randomized assignment to treatment; no confounding due to treatment of other risk factors and no trials which used compounds that were subsequently shown to be toxic, such as *d*-thyroxine and oestrogen (Rossouw *et al.*, 1990).

Baseline mean total cholesterol concentration varied between 6.3 and 7.6 mmol/l. Patients, on the whole, were not entered into the trials until at least three months following myocardial infarction. This is an important consideration as early deaths due to severe myocardial damage would confound treatment effects due to cholesterol lowering.

The results of the meta-analysis are shown in Figure 3.3. Despite the fact that treatment differences were small due to the lack of efficacy or poor tolerability of early drugs (e.g. clofibrate and nicotinic acid) and the use of dietary therapy alone, there was a highly significant reduction in coronary death and non-fatal CHD events. Furthermore there did not appear to be any excess of non-cardiovascular death.

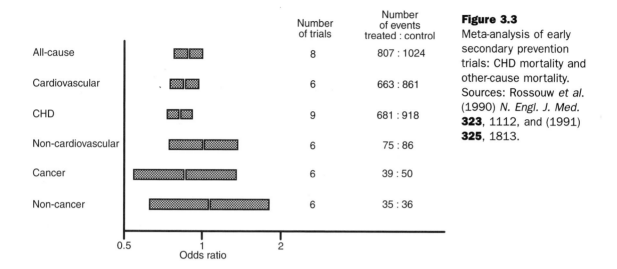

	Number of trials	Number of events treated : control
All-cause	8	807 : 1024
Cardiovascular	6	663 : 861
CHD	9	681 : 918
Non-cardiovascular	6	75 : 86
Cancer	6	39 : 50
Non-cancer	6	35 : 36

Figure 3.3
Meta-analysis of early secondary prevention trials: CHD mortality and other-cause mortality. Sources: Rossouw *et al.* (1990) *N. Engl. J. Med.* **323**, 1112, and (1991) **325**, 1813.

ANGIOGRAPHIC TRIALS

With improvement in angiographic methods for visualizing the coronary arteries and the standardization of these techniques, it has become possible to assess the effect of lipid-lowering therapy on progression and regression of individual coronary artery atherosclerotic plaques. Early studies used a panel of radiologists (blinded to the treatment arm) to score angiograms. More recent studies have used sophisticated computerized techniques which allow increased measurement precision.

Angiographic trials have provided a useful means of assessing the benefits of cholesterol lowering as they can be performed in a relatively short time (two to four years) and on smaller numbers of patients than are required when clinical end-points are studied. The most often quoted measurements in angiographic trials are the minimum lumen diameter and the percentage stenosis. The major angiographic trials are summarized in Table 3.9. To give a flavour of these trials some of them will be discussed in more detail illustrating dietary, combined drug and single drug regimes.

Diet and lifestyle angiographic trials

The Leiden Intervention Trial (LIT) published in 1985 was the first to use quantitative coronary angiography (Barth *et al.*, 1987). This was an uncontrolled study of a low-fat diet (P/S ratio $\geqslant 2$, dietary cholesterol < 100 mg) plus increased exercise (brisk walking for 20 minutes, three times per week) for two years in 39 CHD patients with greater than 50% stenosis in at least one coronary artery. The mean baseline cholesterol was 6.9 mmol/l and LDL cholesterol fell by approximately 10% during the trial period whilst HDL cholesterol increased by 4%. Although these lipoprotein

(a) Summary descriptions for nine reported angiographic lipid-lowering trials: lipid response to treatments

Study	n	Entry requirements	Control regimen[a]	Treatment Regimen	Response LDL	HDL	Years
NHLBI II	143	CAD,LDLD	D	D+R	−31%	+ 8%	5
CLAS I	188	CABG	D (−)	D+R+N	−43%	+37%	2
POSCH	838	MI,CHOL	D	D+PIB±R	−42%	+ 5%	9.7
Lifestyle	48	CAD	U	V+M+E	−37%	− 3%	1
FATS (N+C)				D+R+N	−32%	+43%	2.5
	146	CAD,Apo B	D+R				
FATS (L+C)				D+R+L	−46%	+15%	2.5
CLASII	138	CABG	D	D+R+N	−40%	+37%	4
UC-SCOR	97	FH	U	D+R+N±L	−39%	+25%	2
STARS (D)				D	−16%	0%	3
	90	CAD,CHOL	U				
STARS (D+R)				D+R	−36%	− 4%	3
SCRIP	300	CAD	U	D+(R/N/L/F/)+E,BP	−21%	+13%	4
Heidelberg	113	CAD	U	D+E	−8 %	+ 3%	1

Table 3.9

Summary of recent angiographic trials (Brown et al., 1993). Reproduced with permission

changes were only modest, 46% of patients showed no new lesion growth at two years. Regression was seen in compliant individuals who showed a significant decrease in the LDL cholesterol/HDL cholesterol ratio.

Diet and life style effects have also been studied in the St Thomas Atherosclerosis Regression Study (STARS) (Watts *et al.*, 1992), the Lifestyle Heart Trial (LHT) (Ornish *et al.*, 1990) and the small Heidelberg study (Hambrecht *et al.*, 1993). The intervention adopted in the LHT study of 96 subjects with symptomatic CHD was a very low-fat ($<7\%$ total calories) and cholesterol (12 mg/day) diet together with behavioural modification – yoga, exercise and advice against smoking. Although 96 patients were originally recruited, only 48 completed the study; of these, 41 (22 intervention group and 19 controls) had analysable angiographic film pairs – this is an obvious criticism of the study. Nevertheless a substantial reduction was observed in LDL cholesterol (37%) from a baseline of 3.9 mmol/l in the intervention group compared with 6% in the control group. Apoprotein B also fell by 24% in the intervention group. As a result of the very low-fat and very high-carbohydrate diet, plasma triglyceride rose by 22% in the intervention group.

After one year, repeat quantitative coronary angiography demonstrated a 2.2% reduction in stenosis in the life style intervention group compared with a 3.4% increase in the control group ($P<0.001$). In lesions of greater

(b) Summary of arteriographic outcomes and frequencies of reported clinical events in nine lipid-lowering angiographic trials

Study	Control patients			Treatment patients			% 'Event' reduction[c]
	Progression (%)	Regression (%)	Δ(%S)[b]	Progression (%)	Regression (%)	Δ%S(P)	
NHLBI[II]	49	7	–	32	7	–	33%
CLAS	61	2	–	39	16	–	25%
POSCH (5 years)	65	6	–	37	14	–	35% (62%)[II]
Lifestyle	32	32	+3.4	14	41	–2.2 (0.001)	0 vs. 1
FATS (N+C)				25	39	–0.9 (0.005)	80%[II]
	46	11	+2.1				
FATS (L+C)				22	32	–0.7 (0.02)	70%
CLASII	83	6	–	30	18	–	43%
UC-SCOR	41	13	+0.8	20	33	–1.5 (0.04)	1 vs. 0
STARS (D)				15	38	–1.1 (NS)	69%[II]
	46	4	+5.8				
STARS (D+R)				12	33	–1.9 (0.01)	89%
SCRIP	–	10	–	–	21	–	50%
Heidelberg	42	4	+3.0	20	30	–1.0 (0.05)	
	53	8		26	26		

Apo B, apolipoprotein B ≤ 125 mg/dl; BP, blood pressure therapy; C, colestipol; CABG, coronary artery bypass graft surgery; CAD, coronary artery disease; CHOL, cholesterol > 220 mg/dl; D, diet; E, exercise programme; F, fibrate-type drugs; FH, familial hypercholesterolaemia; HDL, high density lipoprotein; L, lovastatin; LDL, low density lipoprotein > 90th percentile; M, relaxation techniques; MI, myocardial infarction; N, nicotinic acid; PIB, partial ileal bypass; R, resin (colestipol or cholestyramine); U, usual care; V, vegetarian diet < 10% fat

[a] Mean LDL cholesterol response to control regimen, –7%; mean HDL cholesterol response, 0%.

[b] Δ (%S) is usually reported as the average change in percentage stenosis over all the lesions measured per patient. A positive (+) value represents 'progression', negative (–) regression

[c] Events are variably defined in these studies; in general, the frequency of cardiovascular events (death, myocardial infarction, unstable ischaemia requiring revascularization) in control and treated groups are compared using the sometimes sketchy details and definitions provided. Statistical comparison uses a lesion-based method.

[II] Studies for which the reduction in cardiovascular clinical events was statistically significant.

than 50% stenosis there was a 5.3% reduction compared with 2.7% increase in the control group. Although this study is open to criticism it is nevertheless encouraging and does suggest it is possible to make an impact on atherosclerosis with life style measures.

The findings of the LHT were confirmed in the diet limb of the STARS trial, which employed less strict dietary intervention likely to be more acceptable for the majority of patients. The diet consisted of a reduction in

Table 3.9
continued

dietary fat to 27% of daily energy (saturated fat 8–10%; polyunsaturated fat 8%) with a cholesterol intake of 100 mg/1000 kcal. Soluble fibre was increased. Baseline mean cholesterol was 7.2 mmol/l and during the trial period (39 months) was 6.93 in the control and 6.17 mmol/l in the diet group.

This dietary-induced change in plasma cholesterol was associated with an overall progression of coronary narrowing in 15% of patients ($n = 26$ completed) compared with 46% in the control group ($n = 24$ completed) as assessed with quantitative angiography. Furthermore, the proportion of patients who showed an increase in luminal diameter was 38% of the diet group compared with 4% in the control group. The mean absolute width of coronary segments decreased by 0.201 mm in controls compared with an increase in the diet group of 0.003 mm.

Combination drug therapy angiographic trials

The landmark Cholesterol Lowering Atherosclerosis Study (CLAS) was published by the late David Blakenhorn and colleagues (Blakenhorn et al., 1987) The study population consisted of 188 non-smoking, diet-treated men (aged 40–59 years) who had undergone coronary artery bypass grafting. Patients were randomly allocated to receive the anion exchange resin colestipol (30 g/day) and high-dose nicotinic acid (3–12 g/day) or placebo preparations. Additional entry criteria were a total plasma cholesterol between 4.79 and 9.07 mmol/l and a confirmed ability to comply with the proposed study medication, which is notoriously difficult to take. In the intervention group there were impressive reductions in LDL cholesterol (43%) and triglycerides (22%) whilst HDL was substantially increased (37%).

Coronary angiograms at zero and two years were assessed by a panel of experts and a global coronary score was arrived at, based on a comprehensive count of all lesions and an assessment of percentage diameter stenosis for each lesion in native coronary arteries and bypass grafts. The study was completed by 162 patients and in the intervention group there was a significant reduction in the average number of lesions per subject which progressed. In addition, both in native vessels and grafts, new plaque formation was significantly reduced. Using a global score analysis, regression was considered to have occurred in the treated group. This was the first angiographic trial to suggest that regression of atherosclerotic plaques could occur.

A subgroup of 103 patients completed a further two years of follow-up (CLAS-II) during which the lipid and lipoprotein alterations were maintained (Cashin-Hemphill et al., 1990). After four years there were further observed effects on atherosclerosis progression and regression. Plaques remained unchanged ('non-progression') in 52% of patients in the treated group compared with 15% in the placebo group. Regression in native coronaries was observed in 18% in the treated group compared with 6% in the placebo group. Fewer drug-treated patients developed new lesions (14% vs. 40%) in native vessels and in grafts (16% vs. 38%). This highly encouraging study argued for early and vigorous lipid-lowering therapy in coronary bypass graft recipients.

The findings of the CLAS study received considerable support with the publication of the results of the Familial Atherosclerosis Treatment Study (FATS) (Brown *et al.* 1990). The study population consisted of 146 men (< 62 years of age) with a family history of premature cardiovascular disease and angiographically demonstrable CHD with at least one coronary stenosis equal to or greater than 50% or three lesions equal to or greater than 30%. At baseline, apoprotein B levels were greater than 1.25 g/l.

There were three treatment arms: a conventional treatment group which received placebo; a group which received colestipol (30 g/day) and nicotinic acid (4 g/day); and a group which received colestipol (30 g/day) together with the HMG-CoA reductase inhibitor lovastatin (40 mg/day). Patients allocated to the placebo group received colestipol if LDL cholesterol exceeded the 90th percentile for the US population. In the group receiving colestipol and niacin, LDL cholesterol was reduced by 34% and HDL increased by 41%. In the colestipol/lovastatin group, LDL fell by 48% and HDL cholesterol increased by 14%.

Quantitative computer coronary angiography was performed at baseline and at 2.5 years. Nine standard proximal coronary artery segments were analysed and the two principal measures were minimum lumen diameter and percentage stenosis. In the control group, 46% of patients showed definite lesion progression in at least one segment. In the intervention groups, 21% of patients showed progression in the colestipol/lovastatin group and 25% in the colestipol/niacin group. Regression of lesions was observed in 32% of patients taking colestipol and lovastatin and 39% in the colestipol/nicotinic acid group compared with 11% in the control group. These differences were highly statistically significant.

Although an open study, the Specialized Center of Research (SCOR) Familial Hypercholesterolaemia Trial (University of California, San Francisco) is worthy of discussion as the study population consisted of FH heterozygote females as well as males (Kane *et al.*, 1990). Patients were randomized to conventional therapy (diet and low-dose resin) or aggressive therapy with combination drug therapy (colestipol, niacin and lovastatin). Percentage stenosis showed a mean change of + 0.80, indicating progression, compared with − 1.53 in the intervention group, which indicates regression ($P = 0.039$). When males and females were analysed separately, the lesion change was only significant in females.

Single drug angiographic trials

In the pre-HMG CoA reductase era the anion-exchange resin cholestyramine ($n = 59$) was shown to delay lesion progression compared with a diet-treated control group ($n = 57$) in the National Heart Lung Blood Institute (NHLBI) Type II Study – 32% of patients on cholestyramine (LDL reduction 26%) compared with 49% in the control diet group (LDL reduction 5%) (Brensike et al., 1984). Similarly, in the cholestyramine arm of STARS, 12% of patients showed lesion progression compared with 46% in the control group ($P < 0.02$) (Watts et al., 1992).

Several randomized controlled trials have been performed with HMG CoA reductase inhibitors including the Monitored Atherosclerosis Regression Study (MARS) (Blankenhorn et al., 1993) and the Canadian Coronary Atherosclerosis Intervention Trial (CCAIT) (Waters et al., 1994); which used lovastatin. The Multicentre Anti-Atheroma Study (MAAS) used simvastatin (MASS Investigators, 1994), and Pravastatin Limitation of Atherosclerosis in Coronary Arteries (PLAC-1) used pravastatin (Pitt et al., 1995). These studies showed remarkably similar results with the percentage of patients showing progression ranging between 29 and 43% and those showing regression ranging from 10 to 25%. The treatment effects on plasma lipids in these trials were considerable, with LDL reductions of 29–38%.

Much less information is available in relation to fibrate drugs and effects on lesion progression/regression. A small, uncontrolled study involving 21 patients with minor coronary arterial narrowings showed some angiographic changes with diet and fenofibrate over 21 months of treatment. In this study the main lipid effects, as might be expected with a fibrate, were on triglycerides ($- 30\%$) and HDL cholesterol ($+ 19\%$) though total cholesterol also fell ($- 19\%$) (Hehmann et al., 1991).

The first controlled angiographic study using a fibrate has recently been published in *The Lancet*: the Bezafibrate Coronary Atherosclerosis Intervention Trial (BECAIT) (Ericsson et al., 1996). The study population consisted of young male myocardial infarction survivors. Ninety-two patients entered the trial and were randomly allocated to bezafibrate (200 mg tds) or placebo after a three-month period of dietary intervention. Median baseline cholesterol was 6.87 mmol/l in the bezafibrate group and 6.9 mmol/l in the placebo group.

Coronary angiographic data at baseline and at two and five years was available on 81 patients. In the bezafibrate group the minimum lumen diameter, as determined by quantitative angiography, decreased by 0.06 mm compared with 0.17 mm in the placebo group ($P = 0.049$).

These changes are of similar magnitude to those observed in the statin studies and it is of considerable interest that bezafibrate therapy was not associated with a significant reduction in LDL cholesterol, the main effects being on total triglycerides (-31.4%), VLDL triglycerides (-37.17%), VLDL cholesterol (-34.89%) and HDL cholesterol ($+9.18\%$). This study, which needs to be confirmed, raises the intriguing possibility that reduction of triglyceride and increase in HDL may delay progression of atherosclerosis independently of effects on LDL cholesterol.

Programme on the Surgical Control of Hyperlipidaemias (POSCH) study

This unique large angiographic study employed partial ileal bypass surgery to lower cholesterol by interrupting the enterohepatic circulation of bile (Buchwald *et al.*, 1990). Of the 838 men (91%) and women with previous myocardial infarction recruited, 421 were randomized to surgical treatment (5% refused). Coronary angiography was performed at baseline and after 5–10 years. In the non-surgical group some 32% of patients were taking lipid-lowering drugs. LDL cholesterol fell by 38% in the surgical group. Significantly less atherosclerosis progression was observed in the surgical group. Although this form of treatment is now largely redundant, this large trial gave the possibility of examining the effect of prolonged LDL cholesterol lowering on CHD morbidity, which was highly significantly reduced.

Post Coronary Artery Bypass Graft trial

This angiographic trial, which was reported in the *New England Journal of Medicine* in January 1997, is important from several points of view (The Post Coronary Artery Bypass Graft Trial Investigators, 1997). Firstly, it confirms the beneficial effects of lipid-lowering therapy in decreasing the rate of progression of saphenous vein coronary artery bypass grafts in a large group of patients (Table 3.10). In addition (and making this trial a unique contribution), the investigators used a two-by-two factorial design to assign patients to either 'moderate' or 'aggressive' treatment designed to achieve different levels of LDL cholesterol. In the 'aggressive' group, LDL cholesterol concentrations were reduced to between 93 and 97 mg/dl (2.4–2.5 mmol/l) and in the 'moderate' group to between 132 and 136 mg/dl (3.4–3.5 mmol/l). This difference in LDL cholesterol was associated with a significantly lower percentage of grafts showing progression of atherosclerosis. Furthermore there was a reduction in the rate of revascularization procedures in the aggressive treatment group compared with the moderate treatment group.

The results of this study argue for aggressive lowering of LDL cholesterol in patients with established CHD and this is in line with the recommendation of the NCEP in the United States, which has a goal of therapy for such patients of LDL cholesterol less than 100 mg/dl (2.6 mmol/l).

Table 3.10
Post Coronary Artery
Bypass Graft Trial
Investigation (1997)

Study participants:
   1351 men and women (~8%) aged 21–74 years
   with CABG between 1 and 11 years previously.
   Baseline LDL cholesterol, 4 mmol/l.

4.3 year average follow-up; primary angiographic outcome –
   mean percentage per patient of grafts with a decrease of
   0.6 mm or more in lumen diameter.

Two levels of treatment (diet, lovastatin ± cholestyramine) to
   achieve aggressive LDL lowering (2.4–2.5 mmol/l) or
   moderate LDL lowering (3.4–3.5 mmol/l)

Mean percentage of grafts with atherosclerosis progression was
   27% in 'aggressive' group and 39% in moderate group ($P <$
   0.001).

Revascularization procedures reduced by 29% – 6.5% vs. 9.2%,
   ($P = 0.03$).

Clinical events in the angiographic trials

A surprising but gratifying finding in many of the angiographic regression trials was a reduction in clinical events which in some studies, such as POSCH, FATS, STARS, PLAC-1 and BECAIT, was statistically significant. It is important to bear in mind that the trials were not designed to assess impact on clinical events (apart from POSCH). Nevertheless, this finding was impressive given the relatively short time course of the majority of the studies.

It is conceivable that the recorded changes in coronary plaques could explain the decreased number of events, though it seems unlikely that this could be the whole explanation. Brown and colleagues (in an excellent review paper published in *Circulation*) using data from their own FATS study have hypothesized – with considerable supporting evidence – that the explanation for the relatively early impact of lipid lowering on events is likely to be due to stabilization of lipid-rich plaques (Brown *et al.*, 1993). These plaques, which constitute less than 20% of coronary lesions and are generally less than 50% stenosis, have a thin fibrous cap and are prone to rupture, with consequent platelet thrombosis formation and blockage of the artery or at least rapid expansion of the plaque if the thrombosis is incorporated into it. Lipid-lowering therapy may result in mobilization of lipid from these plaques, thus allowing the fibrous cap to thicken.

Stabilization of plaques is a very attractive hypothesis but other mechanisms may play a role. It is now known, for instance, that abnormal arterial endothelial function – which is an important feature of atherosclerotic arteries – can be restored towards normal with lipid-lowering diet and drug therapy (Leung *et al.*, 1993; Treasure *et al.*, 1995; Anderson *et al.*, 1995). The usual technique for demonstrating coronary artery endothelial dysfunction is to instill acetylcholine at the time of angiography. This mediator results in vasodilatation through release of endothelial derived relaxing factor (EDRF) now known to be nitric oxide. In diseased arteries, acetylcholine produces a paradoxical vasoconstriction. Normal responses to acetylcholine in coronary arteries has been restored after 6–12 months of lipid-lowering therapy.

SCANDINAVIAN SIMVASTATIN SURVIVAL STUDY (4S)

The encouraging results of the angiographic trials, taken together with meta-analyses of the early diet and drug secondary prevention trials, suggested overall benefit for cholesterol lowering in secondary prevention. However, for many physicians what was required was a definite clinical trial with sufficient statistical power to determine effects on overall mortality. Fortunately such a landmark trial (4S) was published in 1994 (Scandinavian Simvastatin Survival Study Group, 1994).

The 4S study recruited 4444 patients (872 females) aged 35–70 years with established CHD and total cholesterol concentrations between 5.5 and 8 mmol/l despite 8 weeks' dietary therapy. Originally 7027 patients entered the dietary run-in period and of these 4444 met the entry criteria and were randomized to the HMG-CoA reductase inhibitor simvastatin or placebo.

The impact of cholesterol lowering on overall mortality was the primary end-point of the study and it was necessary to continue the study until 440 deaths had been observed, to meet statistical power calculations. Secondary objectives of the study were the impact on major coronary events, including fatal and non-fatal myocardial infarction and sudden cardiac death. In addition, important tertiary end-points included hospitalization episodes for heart disease, the incidence of cerebrovascular disease and other atherosclerotic diseases and surgical interventions such as coronary artery bypass grafting and angioplasty.

Patients were recruited from 94 cardiac centres throughout the Nordic countries; most had a history of previous myocardial infarction ($\simeq 80\%$) and a minority (20%) had stable angina alone. Excluded from the study were patients at risk of early arrhythmic death including those with unstable angina, congestive heart failure, an enlarged heart or atrial fibrillation and those on anti-arrhythmic therapy.

In the simvastatin group the goal of therapy was a total cholesterol concentration between 3.0 and 5.2 mmol/l. Most patients achieved this goal on 20 mg of simvastatin but 37% of patients required 40 g daily. During the course of the study, substantial differences in lipid and lipoprotein concentrations were maintained with a 35% reduction in LDL cholesterol, an increase in HDL cholesterol of 8% and a reduction in triglyceride of 10%.

The 4S trial finished in August 1994 after the requisite number of deaths had occurred and the median follow-up time was 5.4 years. It is quite remarkable that the vital status of all 4444 patients was available at the end of the trial. The principal results of the study were equally remarkable and had a major impact on the scientific community when they were announced at the American Heart Association in Dallas. There were also front page reports in major newspapers including the *Wall Street Journal* and the *New York Times*.

In the group receiving placebo there were 256 deaths whilst in the simvastatin group there were 182, giving a relative risk of 0.70 (95% confidence intervals 0.59–0.85; P = 0.0003) (Table 3.11). Unfortunately there were insufficient numbers of women recruited to the study to allow effects on overall mortality to be assessed, but a similar reduction in coronary events was observed in women. Furthermore patients aged over 60 years showed similar benefit to younger patients. There was a 37% reduction in the need for revascularization with coronary artery bypass grafting or angioplasty, which is of importance when the cost-effectiveness of cholesterol lowering in secondary prevention is assessed.

A follow-up report from the 4S investigators, and of relevance to clinical practice, has demonstrated that a similar relative risk reduction (35%; 95% confidence intervals 15–50) was observed with simvastatin therapy in those patients in the lowest LDL cholesterol quartile and those in the highest quartile (36%; 95% confidence intervals 19–49) (4S Study Group, 1995). Similar findings were observed for total cholesterol and HDL cholesterol. These findings argue that all CHD patients with total cholesterol concentrations greater than 5.5 mmol/l should be treated.

The analysis of safety parameters in the 4S study provided strong reassurance of the long-term safety and tolerability of simvastatin. This is particularly pleasing given the degree of cholesterol lowering achieved. If cholesterol reduction is associated with increased non-cardiovascular disease, surely it should have been observed in 4S? However, there were no increases in other causes of death. Furthermore, the overall frequency of adverse events was similar in both simvastatin and placebo groups. Significant elevations in liver enzymes (greater than three times upper limit of normal) were seen in only small numbers (Pedersen *et al.*, 1996):

Liver enzyme	Number of patients	
	Simvastatin	Placebo
Aspartate transaminase	20	23
Aminotransferase	33	49

Major increases in creatine phosphokinase (greater than 10 times the upper limit of normal) were seen in seven patients (one on placebo and six on simvastatin). There was only one case of rhabdomyolysis (potentially the most serious side effect of HMG-GoA reductase inhibitors), in a female patient on 20 mg per day simvastatin. The patient recovered when treatment was discontinued.

Details of cancer deaths during the study are shown in Table 3.11. There were no differences in non-fatal cancer cases, with 61 in the placebo and 67 in the simvastatin group.

The 4S authors concluded that the improvement in overall mortality observed with simvastatin therapy was achieved without any suggestion of an increase in non-CHD mortality. Simvastatin therapy was well tolerated and adverse events were similar in the placebo and treated groups. No previously unknown adverse effects were apparent in this trial.

The authors of the 4S study have recently published an important paper dealing with the implications of the study in terms of use of healthcare resources. As discussed elsewhere in this book, the cost of healthcare provision for cardiovascular disease is mammoth ($100 billion per year in the United States) and new therapies do need to be assessed in terms of their cost-effectiveness. In the 4S study there were 1905 hospitalizations (average duration 7.9 days) for coronary disease in 937 patients in the placebo group. In the simvastatin-treated group there were 1403 hospitalizations (average duration 7.1 days) in 720 patients. This is a highly significant difference ($P < 0.0001$). The difference in the number of hospital days was 15 089 versus 9951 (34% reduction; $P < 0.0001$). Based on US prices the reduction in hospital costs over the course of the study (5.4 years) would be equivalent to $3872 per patient. This effectively reduces the cost of simvastatin to $0.28 day, a reduction of 88%. So it can be concluded that the drug cost is largely offset by the reduction in the use of hospital services (Johannesson *et al.*, 1997; Pedersen *et al.*, 1996).

Table 3.11
Scandinavian Simvastatin
Survival Study

Causes of death	Placebo (n = 2223)	Simvastatin (n = 2221)	Relative risk (95% CI)
Definite acute MI	63	30	
Probable acute MI	5	5	
Acute MI not confirmed			
Instantaneous death	39	29	
Death within 1 hour[a]	24	8	
Death within 1–24 hours	15	9	
Death > 24 hours after onset	11	10	
Non-witnessed death[b]	23	13	
Intervention-associated[c]	9	7	
All coronary	189	111	0.58 (0.46–0.73)
Cerebrovascular	12	14	
Other cardiovascular	6	11	
All cardiovascular	207	136	0.65 (0.52–0.80)
Cancer	35	33	
Suicide	4	5	
Trauma	3	1	
Other	7	7	
All non-cardiovascular	49	46	
All deaths	256	182	0.70 (0.58–0,85)

[a] Following acute chest pain, syncope, pulmonary oedema or cardiogenic shock
[b] With no likely non-coronary cause
[c] Coronary death within 28 days of any invasive procedure

CHOLESTEROL AND RECURRENT EVENTS STUDY (CARE)

Preliminary results of this important study were presented at the American College of Cardiology meeting in Orlando, USA, in March 1996 and subsequently published in the *New England Journal of Medicine* (Sacks, *et al.* 1996). CARE is a secondary prevention trial involving 4159 patients (14% female) aged 21–75 years with a myocardial infarction 3–24 months prior to entry to the study. This trial breaks new ground in several respects:

- participants have 'normal' total (< 6.2 mmol/l) and LDL cholesterol concentrations (3.0–4.5 mmol/l);
- 55% of participants had previous coronary artery bypass grafts or PTCA;
- participants were included with left ventricular dysfunction (left ventricular ejection fraction $\geq 25\%$);
- participants were included with entry total triglyceride concentrations up to 4 mmol/l;
- 83% of participants were taking aspirin, 40% beta blockers and 39% calcium antagonists.

Participants were randomly allocated to placebo or the HMG-CoA reductase inhibitor pravastatin, 40 mg/day. Lipid changes observed during the study were LDL cholesterol reduction of 28%, HDL cholesterol increase of 5% and triglyceride reduction of 14%. The mean cholesterol concentration in the pravastatin group was 3.9 mmol/l and the mean LDL cholesterol 2.5 mmol/l

The major end-point of the CARE study was a combination of fatal and non-fatal myocardial infarction and the results are shown in Table 3.12.

Event	Placebo (n = 2078) No.	Placebo (n = 2078) %	Pravastatin (n = 2081) No.	Pravastatin (n = 2081) %	Risk reduction % (95% CI)	P value
CHD death or non-fatal infarction	274	13.2	212	10.2	24 (9–36)	0.003
CHD death	119	5.7	96	4.6	20 (–5–39)	0.10
Non-fatal infarction	173	8.3	135	6.5	23 (4–39)	0.02
Fatal infarction or confirmed non-fatal infarction	207	10.0	157	7.5	25 (8–39)	0.006
Fatal infarction	38	1.8	24	1.2	37 (–5–62)	0.07
CABG or PTCA	391	18.8	294	14.1	27 (15–37)	< 0.001
Unstable angina	359	17.3	317	15.2	13 (–1–25)	0.07
Stroke	78	3.8	54	2.6	31 (3–52)	0.03

Table 3.12
CARE Study (Sacks *et al.*, 1996)

These results are quite remarkable, given the low lipid entry criteria, and give considerable strength to the argument that whatever the cholesterol level, it is 'too high' for the CHD patient and benefit will be observed if it is reduced. When patient subgroups were analysed similar risk reductions were observed in smokers, hypertensives, diabetics and those with low left ventricular ejection fractions. The CARE study will contribute further to the case for secondary prevention. As the population recruited was at lower risk than those in the 4S, it will be important to assess the cost-benefit implications of statin therapy in this study.

Part Two
Screening and Assessment

Screening

A comprehensive plan for CHD prevention in the general population should include both population and individual strategies (Figure 4.1). The population strategy aims to shift the whole population in the direction of lower risk by attention to nutrition, smoking and exercise. The individual or high risk strategy aims to identify and treat those individuals at the higher end of a risk factor distribution in order to reduce the risk of CHD for that individual.

In terms of serum cholesterol, improved nutritional and other life style habits for everyone would result in the mean cholesterol level of the population falling and the risk of CHD being substantially reduced. Some people – for example, those with genetic hyperlipidaemias less responsive to dietary change – would benefit more from being identified and treated individually using the high risk approach. In terms of numbers, however, this would have a relatively small impact on the total number of CHD events occurring in a population, as large numbers exposed to slightly raised cholesterol produce more cases of CHD than small numbers exposed to a high level; this is due to the interaction of other risk factors.

There is no conflict between population and individual strategies, which can run together for maximum preventive effect. They are interactive and mutually supportive. For example, individual advice diffuses out and reinforces public health messages in others, increasing the population effect.

Population strategy

Individual strategy

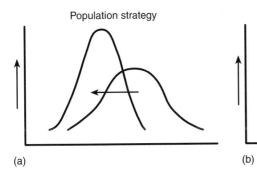

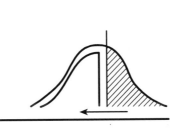

(a)

(b)

Figure 4.1
(a) The population strategy aims to shift the whole population in the direction of lower risk. (b) The high-risk individual strategy aims to identify and treat individuals in the upper part of the distribution.

Population strategy

Since Ancel Keys demonstrated the population differences in the Seven Countries Study, population effects have been seen in several countries – most notably the USA and Australia. Populations tend to behave coherently around the societal norm; so if that norm moves in the direction of health benefit, whole distribution shifts are seen and the large potential of the population strategy is realized. By influencing risk factors in advance, the strategy is seen as radical, rather than the palliative or rescue attempt of the individual approach where risk factors are already established. This has its parallel in famine relief where relief supplies mirror the individual approach while education and agricultural projects reflect the population approach.

The potential of the population strategy for benefit is large but the benefit for the individual is small and those at highest risk may be excluded from benefit at all.

Individual approach

Most health professionals feel comfortable with the individual approach, as the focus is directly on the patient. Patients, too, are better motivated by this traditional personal approach but there are drawbacks. First, the identification of patients at risk requires some sort of screening process, with its attendant difficulties (not least of scale). There are cost implications here, especially as having found 'at risk' individuals there needs to be a management structure to follow them up. By its nature, the individual strategy acts later in the disease process and has more limited potential. It may be more difficult to change the behaviour patterns of people after many years, especially against the societal norm, and there is a risk of labelling people as patients and creating a 'worried well' population.

High risk individuals can be identified in two ways: by **selective** or by **non-selective** (mass) screening.

SELECTIVE VS. NON-SELECTIVE SCREENING

In the UK, selective screening based on the presence of other risk factors is currently recommended (Kings Fund forum, 1989; Standing Medical Advisory Committee, 1990). This recommendation is made on the grounds of cost but is out of step compared with the USA, where ATP II (see p.140) recommends the screening of all adults aged over 20 every 5 years. Other European countries also advocate mass testing – for example, France, where 65% have been tested, and Portugal, 61%, compared with UK, 17%. In these countries it is argued that knowledge of serum cholesterol for an

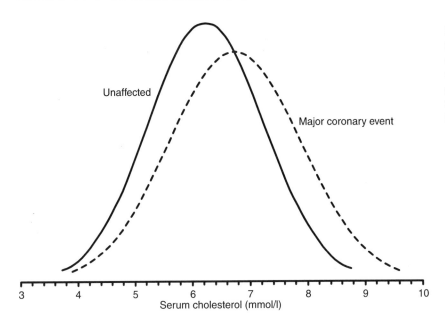

Figure 4.2
Serum cholesterol distribution in 438 men who had a major coronary event and 7252 unaffected men. Source: BRHS.

individual will provide an incentive for change, but this has not been proved and may even be a disincentive if the level is low. Furthermore, serum cholesterol by itself is not necessarily a good screening test and this is shown in BRHS data (Figure 4.2). There is considerable overlap between the curves in Figure 4.2, i.e. a knowledge of serum cholesterol alone does not distinguish between the two populations. Of course, this is due to the action of other risk factors and thus the multifactorial selective approach to screening is favoured. A person is not a cholesterol number but an individual with multiple risk factors present at different levels, of which serum cholesterol is but one.

Counter to this argument is the data from MRFIT, where men with high cholesterol as their only risk factor nevertheless were at greater risk.

In a practice of 10 000 patients, there might be about 45 patients suffering from genetic hyperlipidaemias. Significant numbers of these and other patients with very high cholesterol levels may be missed by even extensive lists of screening criteria including family history, the presence of lipid stigmata, obesity, hypertension and diabetes. It has been estimated that 66% of the population may have to be screened to identify 78% of the people with cholesterol > 6.5 mmol/l.

Selective screening can be adapted to assess patients by risk scores and both the Shaper system (BRHS data) and the Dundee coronary risk-disk have been used for this purpose (pp. 144).

The attraction of selective screening is in its cost-effectiveness. Taking an extreme example, the cost of preventing one myocardial infarction in a 40-year-old-female is 100 times the cost for a 60-year-old male.

HOW MIGHT SCREENING BE ACHIEVED?

Until the time comes when regular checks from cord blood to the grave are standard, there are several available methods.

- Commercial: the advent of portable dry chemistry machines and kits have enabled supermarket and pharmacy testing to be available to the public and this has proved popular. One retail pharmacy chain saw 17 000 patients in four weeks in the UK when it offered this service. Private health insurance agencies also undertake health screening.
- Occupational: it is in industry's interest to maintain its workforce and occupational screening is increasingly common.
- In primary care.

Wherever screening takes place, there are important conditions that must be fulfilled:

- The test should be acceptable to the public and health professionals.
- The test should be accurate and reliable.
- Specialized multifactorial counselling should be available.
- Specific arrangements for management and treatment should be available, of proven efficacy and without adverse effect.

SCREENING IN PRIMARY CARE

The development of the primary care team, with its multidisciplinary, patient-centred approach to multifactorial assessment, makes primary care the ideal setting for risk factor screening. Only primary care can cope with the enormity of the task.

Where there is enthusiasm, significant numbers of patients will respond to the invitation to a screening consultation. Up to 90% will accept if that invitation is made opportunistically while the patient is already at the surgery, even though the consultation will mean a return visit. Systematic screening by postal invitation is much less successful.

Opportunistic screening can take place at any primary care contact and the fact that 70% of patients visit their GP annually and 90–95% over a five-year period means that most of the practice can be screened. As those in social classes IV and V attend more regularly, there is opportunity to address the groups most at need. Spreading the task over years does allow the possibility of tackling the large numbers involved – just screening adults aged 25–60 years means 50% of the practice population. More formal opportunities for screening exist at new patient medicals, well-person checks or designated coronary prevention clinics.

The imposed contractual obligations of health promotion data collection for UK GPs were not successful because the focus was on collecting information for recording purposes rather than using it for risk assessment. Moreover, the central risk factor for CHD prevention – serum cholesterol estimation – was ignored.

Studies of the effectiveness of risk factor intervention ('Health checks') in primary care have been disappointing and this is discussed in Chapter 10.

WHOM TO TEST?

If opportunistic, selective screening is undertaken, cholesterol screening may be offered to patients with:

- a personal history of CHD, peripheral vascular disease or CVA;
- a family history of CHD or PVD (especially before age 55 years) or hyperlipidaemia;
- hypertension;
- diabetes mellitus;
- physical stigmata of hyperlipidaemia;
- obesity (BMI > 28);
- chronic renal disease;
- smoking habits (reflecting the importance of smoking as a major risk factor),
- high Shaper or Dundee risk-disk scores.

The list can be prioritized to reflect patients for whom cholesterol lowering is most effective (cf. British Hyperlipidaemia Association Priorities, p. 220):

- Priority 1:
  - patients with CHD (angina, MI, CABG, angioplasty, etc.);
  - patients with severe family history of lipid stigmata (possibility of genetic disorder);
  - patients with multiple risk factors.

- Priority 2:
  - patients with one risk factor;
  - males with no other risk factors;
  - post-menopausal females.

AGE CONSIDERATIONS

There is no consensus regarding the age at which cholesterol screening can be offered to the population. Even children with heterozygous familial hypercholesterolaemia have abnormal endothelial function and the usual lower limit for screening of 25 years would therefore be inappropriate for cases of genetic hyperlipidaemia. Similarly, the findings in the 4S and CARE intervention trials that patients benefited from secondary prevention up to the ages of 70 and 75, respectively, would cast doubt on the logic of the usual upper age limit of 65 years. Law's meta-analysis (see p. 52) suggested reduced benefit from cholesterol lowering in the elderly but more information is needed and the concept of biological age vs. chronological age is relevant.

FREQUENCY OF TESTING

A reasonable frequency for testing is every five years from age 20–25 years to 60–70 years, according to overall risk. Borderline cases vary from one to five years. For patients on treatment with diet, test initially every three months, then every 6–12 months; for patients on medication, test initially every 6–8 weeks, then every 3–6 months.

WHAT TO TEST?

Fasting has little effect on serum cholesterol levels. In general population screening, where triglyceride estimation is unnecessary, non-fasting specimens are adequate and this makes the test more acceptable to patients.

Unlike total serum cholesterol and HDL levels, the level of triglyceride is affected by meals (chylomicrons from the gut) and in healthy subjects it takes 6–8 hours to produce a steady triglyceride level.

In the high risk patient, such as one with pre-existing CHD, where the clinician requires as much information as possible on the levels of risk factor responsible, it is reasonable to estimate the full fasting profile immediately.

NORMAL VARIATION

We have already seen (Figure 2.10) that serum cholesterol varies within an individual with increasing age. This may not be physiological: South African bushmen on a traditional low fat diet do not show the typical rise in later years demonstrated by those who adopt a more European diet.

Serum cholesterol is subject to a number of influences and these have implications in planning cut-off points for screening programmes and in assessing responses to treatment.

Biological variation

Cholesterol levels vary normally from day to day, week to week and year to year. In a cohort of 14 600 people with repeat cholesterol measurements, the within-person coefficient of variation after one year was 7.4%. A person with a mean value of 6.5 mmol/l would thus have a within-person variation of 7.4% $\times$ 6.5 = about 0.5 mmol/l, i.e. for most of the time (68%) the cholesterol level will fluctuate 0.5 mmol/l either side of 6.5 mmol/l. If one or two other readings are taken (cf. the taking of several readings in the diagnosis of hypertension), the effect of within-person variation is much reduced.

Variation in women

Lipid concentrations vary during the menstrual cycle; both cholesterol and triglycerides tend to peak mid-cycle then fall away towards menstruation. Pregnancy also causes a progressive rise in total cholesterol, HDL and triglycerides, being maximal just before delivery. Serum cholesterol may rise by 1 mmol/l.

Seasonal variation

Serum cholesterol concentrations are highest in the winter and lowest in the summer, varying by 0.5–0.8 mmol/l. This is probably caused by seasonal changes in diet and body weight.

Illness

Illnesses (both major and minor), operations and trauma share the effect of reducing serum cholesterol and raising triglycerides. This effect can be profound and rapid – certainly within 48 hours. Even minor illness such as 'flu can produce a fall that takes three weeks to restore. After major illness or operations, serum cholesterol takes three months to return to previous levels. Reduced cholesterol synthesis is involved and presumably the changes are mediated by catecholamines and corticosteroids. The dangerous significance of this phenomenon lies in misinterpretation of serum cholesterol levels after myocardial infarction or CABG. Blood taken within 24 hours of the event may reflect pre-event levels but sometimes pre-infarction syndromes are operative and sometimes the timing of the event is imprecise.

Several drugs influence lipid levels and they are considered in Chapter 9.

LABORATORY VARIATION AND SAMPLING ERRORS

It is clear that both normal variation and the timing of testing in relation to illness can reduce the interpretive value of serum cholesterol readings. This can be further compounded by sampling errors and inaccuracies in laboratory technique.

When blood is taken the subject should be sitting or lying, preferably after ten minutes rest. Venous blood should be taken avoiding haemostasis

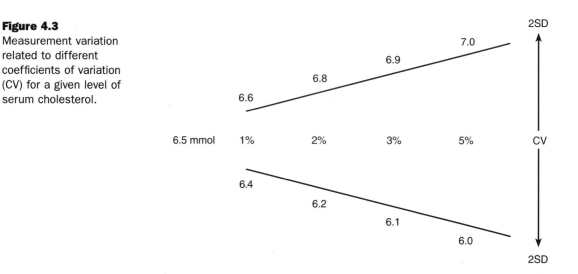

Figure 4.3
Measurement variation related to different coefficients of variation (CV) for a given level of serum cholesterol.

(preferably not using a tourniquet) and avoiding haemolysis (cholesterol leaks from ruptured red cell membranes).

Nowadays, laboratories use automated enzymic methods for lipid estimations. Figure 4.3 shows the measurement variation related to different coefficients of variation for a given level of serum cholesterol. Modern laboratories should achieve coeffcents of variation less than 3% and many approach 2%. This measurement variation emphasizes the need for repeated testing, particularly in the diagnostic and assessment settings, and makes a mockery of those laboratories that report serum cholesterol levels to two decimal places.

Triglyceride levels are even more inaccurate, being subject to wider natural variation within individuals and of course being affected by the timing of the last meal. HDL cholesterol levels are also subject to variation, the more so as different laboratories tend to use different measurement kits.

Clearly, if the basic elements of the lipid profile are so variable, it follows that calculated elements such as LDL and ratios involving HDL are also affected. The inaccuracies surrounding HDL measurement have cast doubt on the usefulness of ratios, particularly when values of HDL are low. Ratios are helpful in the assessment of menopausal women where HDL values are often high.

NEAR SITE TESTING

The feasibility of mass near site testing increased with the development of compact measurement machines such as the Reflotron or the Lipotrend C. Costing several thousand pounds and weighing 5.5 kg, they do not rival the sphygmomanometer as a cheap and convenient instrument. Both machines use a dry reagent strip with a drop of venous or capillary blood. The value is read by reflectance photometry and takes five minutes to complete, allowing perhaps 50 tests in a day. Quality control is achieved using strips to check the optical system and external assessment using control sera is recommended.

In 1989, Broughton estimated the coefficient of variation in three surveys to be 5.5%, worsening with poor technique (e.g. not allowing alcohol from the swab to dry). Unfortunately, this means it is impossible to distinguish between serum cholesterol samples as far apart as 5.2–6.5 mmol/l. Other authors have claimed CVs of 3–5%.

Doubts over accuracy demand cautious interpretation and near site testing may only be useful as a crude screening tool. In the future, however, such testing is likely to improve and direct measurements of HDL and LDL will be available.

The clinician can be forgiven for feeling downhearted about the validity of serum cholesterol readings. As with any diagnostic technology, the problem is one of balancing false positives (patients initiating treatment unnecessarily) and false negatives (patients receiving false reassurance). Only repeated testing and careful consideration in the assessment phase (Chapter 6) can mitigate this.

Diagnosis

5

The interpretation of blood lipid concentrations should not be performed in isolation. The results should be applied to the individual in the knowledge of other risk factors and concurrent diseases, the family history and clinical evaluation, as discussed in Chapter 6.

There has been a tendency to see the results of blood lipid investigations as diagnoses in themselves – hypercholesterolaemia, hypertriglyceridaemia, etc. This is unfortunate and probably relates to the first classification of lipid disorders proposed by Fredrickson and colleagues at the National Institutes of Health in the United States and later adopted by the WHO (Beaumont *et al.*, 1970). This classification was based solely on laboratory parameters using a combination of cholesterol and triglyceride measurements and lipoprotein electrophoresis (Table 5.1).

It is likely that many readers will remember struggling to get to grips with the various types of hyperlipidaemia the evening before examinations, instantly forgetting them thereafter. Although now largely abandoned, there is no doubt that this classification enabled much progress to be made in understanding lipoprotein metabolism and the biochemical basis of the hyperlipidaemias.

New ways of classifying hyperlipidaemias have been developed because the WHO classification does not provide insight into the underlying diagnosis or pathophysiological abnormalities. Type II hyperlipidaemia, for example, may be due on the one hand to hypothyroidism (an important secondary cause of hypercholesterolaemia) and on the other to an inborn error of cholesterol metabolism such as familial hypercholesterolaemia. In addition, HDL is not considered in the WHO classification.

The most useful classification of blood lipid disorders is into primary and secondary dyslipidaemias. Dyslipidaemia is preferable to hyperlipidaemia because qualitative as well as quantitative abnormalities occur, and in the case of HDL the abnormality is often low concentrations.

Most laboratories will provide cholesterol and triglyceride concentrations, but unfortunately some laboratories still resist clinicians' requests for HDL cholesterol measurements. It is difficult to understand this attitude. In defence, some laboratories claim budgetary problems, but perhaps the real reason is that the measurement of HDL cholesterol is still a manual method and therefore inconvenient for the laboratory. It is hoped that the introduction of direct methods will make HDL cholesterol concentrations easier to obtain.

Without a full lipid profile including HDL, the situation is akin to assessing a patient with a low haemoglobin without access to red cell

Table 5.1
WHO classification of hyperlipidaemias and hyperlipoproteinaemias

Type	Appearance of serum	Cholesterol	Lipids Triglycerides	Fasting chylomicrons
I	'Cream layer'; clear infranatant	Normal or ↑	Greatly ↑	↑
IIa	Clear	↑	Normal	Absent
IIb	Clear or faintly turbid	↑	↑	Absent
III	Usually turbid, may be also faint 'cream layer'	↑	↑	Present, may be ↑
IV	Usually turbid	Normal or ↑	↑	Absent
V	'Cream layer'; turbid infranatant	Normal or ↑	Greatly ↑	↑

Type	Lipoprotein pattern LDL	VLDL	HDL	Electrophoretic mobility
I	Normal or ↓	Mildly ↑, normal or ↓	↓	Chylomicron at origin
IIa	↑	Normal or ↓	Normal or ↓	β band ↑
IIb	↑	↑	Normal or ↓	β band ↑, pre-β band ↑
III	Density 1.006[a] – 1.019 ↑ Density 1.019–1.063 ↓	↑[b]	Normal or ↓	'Broad β' band
IV	Normal or ↓	↑	Normal or ↓	Pre-β band ↑
V	Normal or ↓	↑	Usually ↓	Chylomicrons and pre-β band ↑

[a] Intermediate density lipoproteins. (Beaumont *et al.*, 1970, Classification of hyperlipidaemias and hyperlipoproteinaemias, *Bulletin of the World Health Organisation* **43**, 891–915)
[b] 'Floating' β-lipoproteins – density <1.006 g/ml with β-electrophoretic mobility.

morphology or measures of haematinics. HDL cholesterol is important in its own right in helping better to determine individual CHD risk. Furthermore, with knowledge of the full profile it is possible to calculate LDL cholesterol – which is the major therapeutic target in most patients. LDL cholesterol is determined using the Friedewald formula (Friedewald *et al.*, 1972) (all concentrations in mmol/l):

$$\text{LDL cholesterol} = \text{total cholesterol} - \text{HDL cholesterol} - \frac{\text{total triglyceride}}{2.19}$$

The function, total triglyceride/2.19, provides an estimate of VLDL cholesterol based on the usual lipid composition of this lipoprotein. It is reasonably accurate when total triglyceride levels are below 4.5 mmol/l, but the formula is unreliable when triglycerides are high. In this situation LDL cholesterol can be measured after removal of triglyceride-rich lipoproteins by ultracentrifugation, which is available in specialist centres. It is best to obtain at least two and preferably three lipid profiles before making long-term decisions on management, particularly before deciding on drug therapy.

Most laboratories report biochemical parameters as locally determined reference ranges. These are derived from measurement of the particular analyte in many samples (often obtained from blood donors) with calculation of the mean together with a measure of the distribution of the measurements around the mean. The reference range is often reported as the mean ± 1 or 2 standard deviations.

This traditional method of reporting reference ranges is inappropriate for lipid measurements. It is useful to report results in relation to desirable lipid levels in terms of CHD risk. Many laboratories have adopted this approach and emphasize on the report form the importance of assessing overall risk. Taking into account major findings from epidemiological studies relating increasing cholesterol to CHD, several cut-points have evolved somewhat arbitrarily but have received general acceptance by national and international bodies.

Countries where the standard unit is mmol/l are at a disadvantage as the cut-point levels are often not round numbers. This is because the original cut-points were defined as round numbers in mg/dl which, when converted to mmol/l, are no longer round numbers. Thus the desirable level of cholesterol is taken as below 200 mg/dl. This becomes 5.2 when converted to mmol/l. Similarly 300 mg %, the cut-point for severe hypercholesterolaemia, becomes 7.8 mmol/l.

The cut-points adopted by the National Cholesterol Education Program in the United States (National Cholesterol Education Program, 1993), the European Atherosclerosis Society (International Task Force, 1992) and the

Table 5.2
Guidelines

> **(a) National Instututes of Health, USA, Adult Treatment Panel II recommendations: summary of ATPII guidelines[a]**
>
> | Patient category | LDL initiation level | LDL goal |
> |---|---|---|
> | | Dietary therapy | |
> | CHD risk factors < 2 | ≥ 4.1 mmol/l | < 4.1 mmol/l |
> | CHD risk factors ≥ 2 | ≥ 3.4 mmol/l | < 3.4 mmol/l |
> | With CHD | > 2.6 mmol/l | ≤ 2.6 mmol/l |
> | | Drug treatment | |
> | CHD risk factors < 2 | ≥ 4.9 mmol/l | < 4.1 mmol/l |
> | CHD risk factors ≥ 2 | ≥ 4.1 mmol/l | < 3.4 mmol/l |
> | With CHD | ≥ 3.4 mmol/l | ≤ 2.6 mmol/l |
>
> CHD risk factors:
> Positive
>   Age (years)
>   Men > 45
>   Women ≥ 55 or premature menopause without oestrogen replacement therapy
>   Family history of premature CHD
>   Smoking
>   Hypertension
>   HDL cholesterol < 0.9 mmol/l
>   Diabetes
>
> Negative
>   HDL cholesterol > 1.6 mmol/l
>
> [a] Source: Expert Panel Second Report. Detection, evaluation and treatment of high blood cholesterol in adults (Adult Treatment Panel II), National Institutes of Health, Publication No. 93–3095, 1993. *Circulation* (1994) **89**, 1329–1445.

British Hyperlipidaemia Association (Betteridge *et al.*, 1993) are shown in Table 5.2 (a, b, c) for comparison. A major difference is that American guidelines are based on LDL cholesterol, which is more widely available and understood in that country. It is hoped that in future the European bodies will also adopt this policy.

Cut-points for hypertriglyceridaemia also suffer from the mg/dl to mmol/l conversion. The cut-point 200 mg/dl for significant hypertriglyceridaemia becomes 2.3 mmol/l (Table 5.3).

Table 5.2
Guidelines *continued*

(b) European Atherosclerosis guidelines: management of hypercholesterolaemia[a]

Therapeutic group	Conservative measures (weight loss, lipid-lowering diet)	Drugs (based on LDL cholesterol)
Cholesterol 5.2–6.5 mmol/l LDL cholesterol 3.5–4.5 mmol/l	Effective in majority	Only in CHD or very high risk and unresponsive to diet
Cholesterol 6.5–7.8 mmol/l LDL cholesterol 4.5–5.5 mmol/l	Need close dietary compliance Most respond adequately	CHD or high risk if LDL > 3.5 mmol/l and unresponsive to diet
Cholesterol 7.8 mmol/l LDL cholesterol > 5.5 mmol/l	Needs close dietary compliance Three-month trial	Justified even in absence of other risk factors in genetic forms of hypercholesterolaemia

Factors affecting risk:
Modifiable factors: hypertension, cigarette smoking, diabetes mellitus, obesity, low HDL cholesterol, high fibrinogen
Other factors: personal history of CHD, family history of premature vascular disease, male sex, post-menopausal women
[a] Source: International Task Force (1992) Prevention of coronary heart disease: scientific background and new clinical guidelines. Recommendations of the European Atherosclerosis Society. *Nutrition, Metabolism and Cardiovascular Disease*, **2**, 113–156.

HDL cholesterol levels are now included in most guidelines and low levels (< 0.9 mmol/l) are regarded as an important CHD risk factor. Conversely, a high HDL cholesterol concentration (> 1.6 mmol/l) is regarded as a negative risk factor.

Some laboratories measure apoprotein levels for the assessment of dyslipidaemic patients. The usefulness of apoprotein E phenotyping is discussed in the section on remnant particle disease, and the identification of C-II deficiency in the section on familial chylomicronaemia, later in this chapter. These estimations are available in specialist lipid referral centres.

Table 5.2
Guidelines *continued*

(c) British Hyperlipidaemia Association guidelines: priorities and action limits for lipid-lowering drug therapy in diet-resistant subjects[a]

Priority	Subject category	Cholesterol (mmol/l)	
		Total	LDL
First	Patients with existing CHD, or post-CABG, angioplasty or cardiac transplant	> 5.2	> 3.4
Second	Patients with multiple risk factors or genetically determined hyperlipidaemia, e.g. FH	> 6.5	> 5.0
Third	Males with asymptomatic hypercholesterolaemia	> 7.8	> 6.0
Fourth	Post-menopausal females with asymptomatic hypercholesterolaemia	> 7.8 and HDL ratio < 0.2	> 6.0

The aim of cholesterol lowering should be an LDL cholesterol < 3.4 mmol/l in the presence of CHD and < 4.1 mmol/l in the absence of CHD.

[a] Source: Betteridge, D.J. *et al.* (1993) Management of hyperlipidaemia: guidelines of the British Hyperlipidaemia Association. *Postgraduate Medical Journal*, **69**, 359–369.

The question arises as to whether routine laboratories should adopt other apoprotein measurements to help determine CHD risk such as apoprotein A-I (the major HDL protein) and apoprotein B (the major LDL protein). These measurements are relatively easy to perform using automated immunochemical methods. However, do they add to or improve on the information provided by the simple lipid profile? The evidence so far from prospective epidemiology studies that have incorporated these assessments is that they do not.

Measurement of apoprotein B may be clinically useful in certain situations. In a patient with CHD and an apparently normal cholesterol concentration, apoprotein B measurement may be high, as discussed in the section on familial combined hyperlipidaemia. Apoprotein B is also helpful in the assessment of CHD risk in the hypertriglyceridaemic patient with a relatively normal cholesterol concentration.

Therapeutic group	Conservative measures	Drugs
Triglyceride 2.3–4.6 mmol/l LDL cholesterol < 3.5 mmol/l	Reduction of overweight Attention to underlying causes Lipid-lowering diet Appropriate aerobic exercise	Considered if HDL low in CHD or high-risk patients[a]
Triglyceride > 4.5 mmol/l LDL cholesterol < 3.5 mmol/l	Reduction of overweight Attention to underlying causes Lipid-lowering diet Appropriate aerobic exercise	Persistent severe (> 6–8 mmol/l) hypertrigly-ceridaemia unresponsive to diet

[a] Factors affecting risk
Modifiable factors: hypertension, cigarette smoking, diabetes mellitus, obesity, low HDL cholesterol, high fibrinogen.
Other factors: Personal history of CHD, family history of premature vascular disease, male sex, post-menopausal women.

Table 5.3
Guidelines for hypertriglyceridaemia (International Task Force for Prevention of Coronary Heart Disease, 1992)

The importance of lipoprotein(a) as a risk factor in the presence of hypercholesterolaemia has been discussed elsewhere (p. 19). Whether its routine measurement will help in clinical practice remains an unresolved question. In addition there is an urgent need for a generally accepted standardization of its measurement. The authors do use lipoprotein(a) measurement in certain groups of patients for further assessment of CHD risk. In young adults with heterozygous FH, particularly females, a high lipoprotein(a) measurement would point to more aggressive treatment. Similarly in primary prevention a high lipoprotein (a) concentration may tip the balance in favour of drug treatment.

The epidemiological studies that link increasing fibrinogen to CHD risk are convincing and although not a 'lipid factor' the authors certainly include this parameter in their CHD risk assessment.

There is no doubt that new biochemical and genetic measurements to identify vascular risk more precisely will be developed in the future. Important candidates would be oxidized LDL, small dense LDL and remnant particles.

Secondary dyslipidaemias

Faced with significantly abnormal lipid concentrations the clinician must, first of all, exclude possible secondary causes of dyslipidaemia. The more common secondary causes together with the resulting lipid abnormalities are shown in Table 5.4. Additional biochemical tests may be needed to exclude or confirm these disorders. Common secondary causes presenting to the primary care physician are hypothyroidism, obesity, non-insulin-dependent diabetes, high alcohol intake and some drug therapies.

Although hypothyroidism is most commonly linked to hypercholesterolaemia due to increased LDL cholesterol concentrations, any dyslipidaemia can occur in this condition. The clinician should have a low threshold for requesting a TSH estimation. Several secondary and tertiary referrals to the Lipid Clinic have required extremely tactful letters to referring physicians. One lady's diet-resistant hypercholesterolaemia was attributed to the fact that she worked in a fish and chip shop, but it responded to thyroxine therapy following the diagnosis of hypothyroidism. A referral from a consultant colleague posed a potentially difficult clinical problem: a man with CHD and hypercholesterolaemia was intolerant of statin drugs because

Table 5.4
Secondary causes of dyslipidaemia

Cause	Cholesterol	Triglyceride	HDL
		Effects	
Diabetes mellitus			
NIDDM		↑	↓
IDDM: poor control		↑	↓
good control		↓	↑
Hypothyroidism	↑		
Obesity	↑	↑	
Alcohol abuse		↑	
Chronic renal failure	↑	↑	
Nephrotic syndrome	↑ ±	↑	
Cholestasis	↑		
Acute hepatocellular disease	↑	↑	↓
Gout		↑	
Anorexia nervosa	↑		
Bulimia		↑	
Pregnancy		↑	
Immunoglobin excess	↑	↑	

of aches and pains. He was hypothyroid clinically as well as biochemically.

Dyslipidaemia often occurs in association with other risk factors that require drug therapy, such as hypertension. Some commonly used anti-hypertensives may adversely affect blood lipid levels. In patients requiring multiple drug therapy, care should be taken in the choice of anti-hypertensive agent for the dyslipidaemic patient.

Other drugs may have adverse effects on blood lipid concentrations – particularly the corticosteroids, which can increase both cholesterol and triglyceride (Table 5.5). A drug-induced dyslipidaemia seen more frequently follows the increasing use of isotretinoin compounds for severe acne. These drugs may produce a mixed dyslipidaemia, often accompanied by a reduction in HDL cholesterol. The effects of these drugs (as with most other drugs that adversely affect lipids) are more pronounced in those patients with underlying lipid disorders and other secondary causes such as obesity, excess alcohol and diabetes. The dose of isotretinoin may have to be reduced if the dyslipidaemia fails to respond to dietary measures.

Abnormal liver function tests with modest abnormalities in transaminases and alkaline phosphatase in patients with mixed dyslipidaemia are more likely to be secondary to the dyslipidaemia than a cause of it. Mixed dyslipidaemia, particularly when there is associated glucose intolerance or frank diabetes, is often associated with fatty liver which is readily seen on ultrasound. These changes resolve when the dyslipidaemia is treated. Liver abnormalities resulting in secondary hypercholesterolaemia are usually asso-ciated with cholestasis such as primary biliary cirrhosis and sclerosing cholangitis.

Table 5.5
Effects of drugs on lipids, lipoproteins and aproproteins

Drug	Cholesterol	Triglyceride	LDL-C	HDL-C	Apo A-1	Apo B
Retinoids	↑ 25%	↑ 100%	↑ 35%	↓ 30%	→	↑ 35%
Cyclosporin	↑ 40%	↑ 160%	↑ 60%	↓ 15%	↓ 15%	↑ 80%
Phenytoin	→↑	→	↓ 20%	↑ 30%	↑ 10%	↑ 15%
Phenobarbitone	↑ 10%	→	↑ 20%	↑ 40%	↑ 10%	↑ 15%
Carbamazepine	↑ 0–15%	↑ 15%	↑ 15%	↑ 15%	↑10%	→↑
Valproate	↓ 10%	→	↓ 15%	→	→	→
Heparin		↓ 35%				
β agonists	→	→	→	↑ 10%		
Oestrogens	*	↑	↓	↑	↑	↓
Progestogens	*	→↑	→↑	↓	↓	
Corticosteroids	↑	↑	↑	↑		

* Effects depend on type of oestrogen and progestogen and route of administration.

Primary dyslipidaemias

Having excluded secondary dyslipidaemias on clinical grounds and, where necessary, with further laboratory analyses, it is important to make a diagnosis of the primary disorder where possible (Table 5.6). The clinical relevance of this process will become apparent following discussion of the various conditions. Diagnosis of the different dyslipidaemias carries different implications for CHD risk, family screening and genetic counselling, and clinical management.

The underlying biochemical and genetic mechanisms are well understood in some of the primary disorders such as familial hypercholesterolaemia and dysbetalipoproteinaemia (remnant particle disease, type III dyslipidaemia). In others, such as familial combined hyperlipidaemia, much still needs to be learned.

FAMILIAL HYPERCHOLESTEROLAEMIA (FH)

FH is the best understood of the primary dyslipidaemias. Studies of FH patients have demonstrated the importance of raised cholesterol as a critical CHD risk factor but have also enabled major advances to be made in the understanding of cholesterol metabolism. Experiments on cultured skin fibroblasts from homozygous FH patients helped in the discovery of the LDL receptor by the Nobel laureates Michael Brown and Joseph Goldstein in Dallas (Brown and Goldstein, 1986).

Inheritance
FH is an autosomal dominant condition which in the heterozygous state affects approximately 1 : 500 in European populations. In some populations, such as the Lebanese and South Africans of Dutch descent, it is more common – approximately 1 : 100.

A typical family tree is shown in Figure 5.1 Homozygotes or compound heterozygotes are fortunately extremely rare, at approximately one in a million. The vertical transmission through three generations is readily apparent, with roughly equal numbers of offspring affected and an equal sex distribution.

Pathophysiology
The genetic abnormality lies in the LDL receptor gene resulting in either absent or defective LDL receptor activity. Over 400 different mutations in the LDL receptor gene resulting in the FH phenotype have so far been described, and undoubtedly many more remain to be discovered. Halving of

Disease	WHO phenotype	Typical lipid levels (mmol/l)	Lipoproteins	CHD risk	Pancreatic risk	Possible clinical signs
Polygenic hypercholesterolaemia	IIa	Chol 6.5–9, trig < 2.3	LDL ↑	+	–	Xanthelasma, corneal arcus
Familial hypercholesterolaemia	IIa	Chol 7.5–16, trig < 2.3	LDL ↑	+++	–	Tendon xanthoma, arcus, xanthelasma
Familial defective apoprotein B_{100}	IIa	Chol 7.5–16, trig < 2.3	LDL ↑	+++	–	Tendon xanthoma, arcus, xanthelasma
Familial combined hyperlipidaemia	IIa, IIb, IV or V	Chol 6.5–10, trig 2.3–12	LDL ↑ VLDL ↑ HDL ↓	++	–	Arcus, xanthelasma
Remnant particle disease	III	Chol 9–14, trig 9–14	IDL ↑	+++	±	Palmar striae, tuberoeruptive xanthomata
Familial hypertriglyceridaemia	IV, V	Chol 6.5–12, trig 10–30	VLDL ↑ Chylomicrons ↑	?	++	Eruptive xanthomata, lipaemia retinalis, hepatosplenomegaly
Lipoprotein lipase deficiency	– I	Chol < 6.5, trig 10–30	Chylomicrons ↑	–	+++	Eruptive xanthomata, lipaemia retinalis, hepatosplenomegaly
High HDL	–	HDL chol > 2.0	HDL ↑	–	–	–

Chol, cholesterol; trig, triglycerides.
International Task Force for Prevention of Coronary Heart Disease, 1992, Prevention of coronary heart disease: scientific background and new clinical guidelines. Recommendation of the European Atherosclerosis Society. *Nutrition, Metabolism and Cardiovascular Disease*, **2**, 113–156).

Table 5.6
Primary dyslipidaemias

Figure 5.1
Typical family tree
demonstrating inheritance
of familial
hypercholesterolaemia. MI
= myocardial infarction.
Source: Mann, J.L. (1989)
Lipid Rev. **3**, 33.

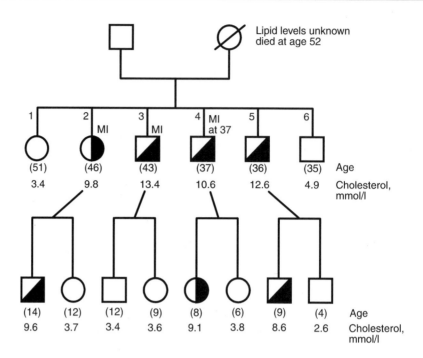

normal receptor function in the heterozygote results in LDL cholesterol
levels that are increased two- to three-fold. The plasma half-life of LDL is
also prolonged. In FH homozygotes, LDL cholesterol levels may be elevated
six-fold.

Clinical features

The clinical stigmata of FH are often striking and sometimes spectacular.
Corneal arcus (Plate 2) and xanthelasma (Plate 3) can occur in young adults
but the clinical hallmark is the presence of tendon xanthomata (Plate 4).
These cholesterol deposits are seen commonly in the Achilles tendon and in
extensor tendons over the back of the hands. Subperiosteal xanthomata also
occur on the elbow and at the tibial tuberosity.

The development of xanthomata is a function of age; in some series 70%
of patients have xanthomata by the age of 30 years and 90% by the age of
40 years. Xanthomata are usually asymptomatic but occasionally tenosyno-
vitis occurs, particularly in the ankles. The most important feature of
xanthomata (and the reason for their multiple illustration in this book) is
their lack of recognition by physicians and surgeons. Our favourite explanation given to one patient was that the xanthomata on the back of the hand

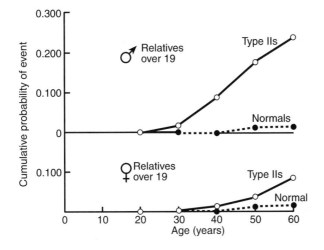

Figure 5.2
Premature atherosclerosis in familial hypercholesterolaemia: cumulative probability of myocardial infarction or coronary heart disease in family members with FH or normal lipid concentrations. Source: Stone *et al.* (1974) *Circulation* **49**, 476.

were as a result of rugby playing injuries! In FH homozygotes, quite bizarre xanthomata may be present with orange-yellow deposits in the skin (planar xanthomata) over the buttocks, knees and hands and between the fingers.

The most important clinical feature of FH is the development of premature and extensive atherosclerosis. Although the contribution to overall CHD within the population is small, the effect can be devastating in individual families (Figure 5.2 and Table 5.7). In the early observational studies the average age of onset of CHD in male heterozygotes was 43 years and in females 53 years. In homozygotes symptomatic CHD can occur in childhood and very few survive past the age of 30 years. In a prospective study of FH heterozygotes in the UK a hundred-fold increased risk of death was observed (Scientific Steering Committee, 1991).

Age (years)	Coronary heart disease		All causes	
	SMR	95% Confidence intervals	SMR	95% Confidence intervals
20–39	9686[a]	(3670–21 800)	902[a]	(329–1950)
40–59	519[a]	(224–1020)	253[a]	(134–432)
60–74	44	(1–244)	69	(22–160)
20–74	386[a]	(210–639)	183[b]	(117–273)

Source: Scientific Steering Committee, Simon Broome FH Register, 1991, *Br. Med. J.*, 303, 893.
[a] $P < 0.001$
[b] $P < 0.01$

Table 5.7
Standardized mortality ratios (SMR) for coronary heart disease and all causes in prospective follow-up study of patients with familial hypercholesterolaemia

Diagnosis

The diagnosis of FH is an important one to make. The high risk of premature CHD in the absence of other risk factors warrants aggressive lipid-lowering therapy, often with a combination of drugs. It is the authors' practice to undertake regular non-invasive testing for silent ischaemia in FH heterozygotes, with stress ECGs every one to two years. This is particularly important if the age of onset of CHD is early in a particular family.

Family screening is mandatory in FH. The majority of heterozygotes remain unidentified and untreated. Screening the families of affected individuals provides a pick up rate of approximately 50%, given the autosomal dominant transmission. The condition exhibits complete phenotypic expression in children and it is our practice to advise testing of children around the age of 5–10 years.

The diagnosis is straightforward when there is a strong family history of premature CHD together with high cholesterol and xanthomata in the index case (Table 5.8). However, not all individuals have xanthomata and family history may be non-contributory. Here the primary care physician is in an excellent position to help in the diagnosis by family screening. As other hyperlipidaemias do not tend to be expressed in childhood, the finding of high cholesterol in children and adolescents strongly points to the diagnosis of FH. A simple, non-fasting cholesterol is usually all that is required. Although special laboratories can now undertake LDL receptor analysis this is not yet helpful in routine practice as there is such a large

Table 5.8
Diagnostic criteria for heterozygous familial hypercholesterolaemia

Definite FH	Possible FH
(a) Child under 16: total cholesterol above 6.7 mmol/l or LDL cholesterol above 4.0 mmol/l; adult; total cholesterol above 7.5 mmol/l or LDL cholesterol above 4.9 mmol/l	
Plus	Plus
(b) Tendon xanthomata in patient or relative (parent, child, grandparent, sibling, aunt, uncle)	(b) Family history of myocardial infarction below age 50 in 2nd degree relative, or below 60 in 1st degree relative
Or	Or
(c) DNA-based evidence of an LDL receptor mutation	(c) Family history of raised cholesterol in 1st degree relative or a history of cholesterol above 7.5 mmol/l in 2nd degree relative

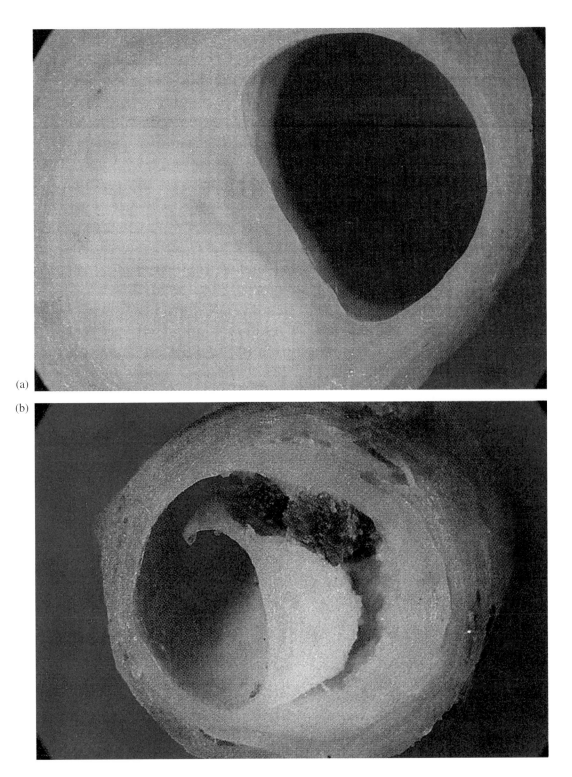

Plate 1 (a) Human coronary atherosclerotic plaque. The lipid-rich core is separated from the lumen by a fibrous cap. Opposite the plaque is an arc of normal vessel wall. (b) Coronary atherosclerotic plaque disruption. The fibrous cap is torn and projects into the arterial lumen and thrombus is present in the plaque core. (Reproduced with permission from Davies, M.J. 1996 *Circulation*, **94**, 2013–20.)

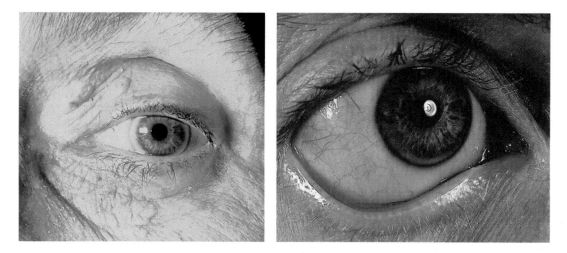

Plate 2 Corneal arcus.

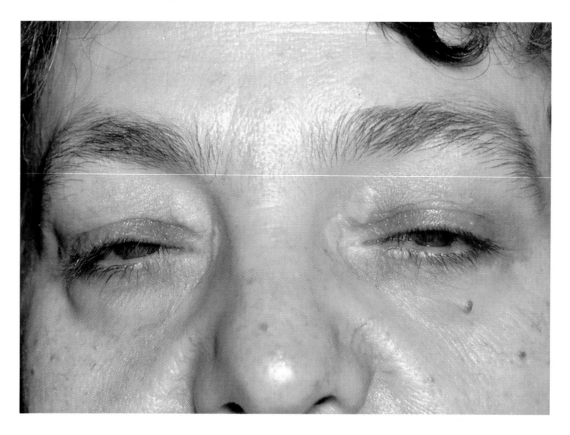

Plate 3 Xanthelasmata.

(a)

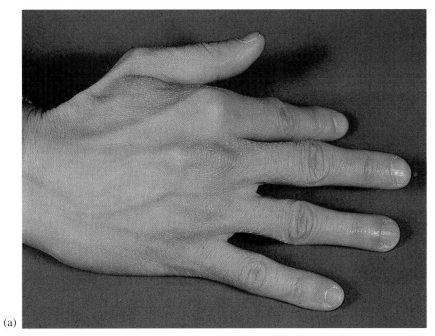

(b)

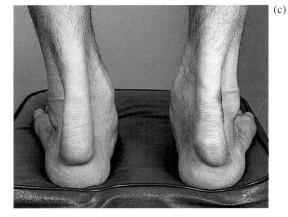

(c)

Plate 4 Tendon Xanthomata in (a) extensor tendons of hand, (b) patellar tendon and subperiosteal xanthomata and (c) Achilles tendon.

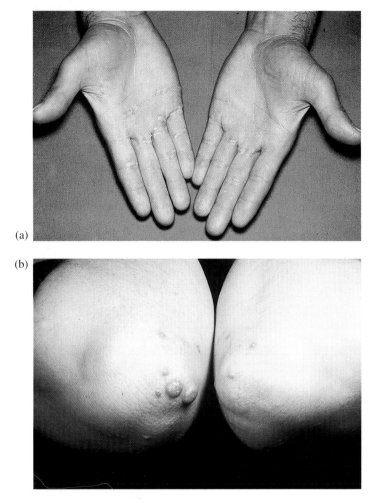

(a)

(b)

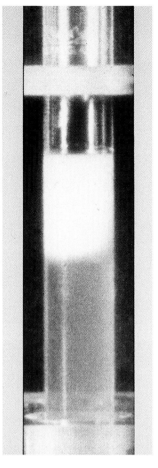

Plate 5 Clinical stigmata of type III dyslipoproteinaemia (a) palmar xanthomata; (b) tubero-eruptive xanthomata.

Plate 6 Characteristic cream layer of Type I hyperlipidaemia plasma. The sample was placed in the refrigerator overnight.

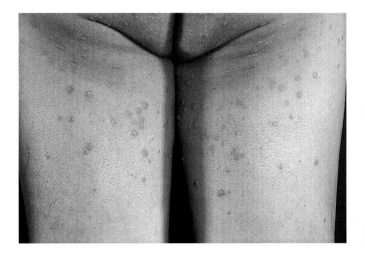

Plate 7 Eruptive xanthomata.

number of mutations and many remain to be identified. In a family with a known mutation, DNA testing for the receptor gene defect is quick and effective and can be performed on saliva as well as blood samples.

FAMILIAL DEFECTIVE APOPROTEIN B (FDB)

Familial defective apoprotein B, first described in 1986 (Vega and Grundy, 1986; Innerarity *et al.*, 1990), can produce a clinical phenotype indistinguishable from familial hypercholesterolaemia but defective clearance of LDL is due to a mutation in apoprotein B (apoB) ligand rather than the receptor. The mutation at codon 3500, which is inherited as an autosomal dominant, leads to the substitution of glutamine for arginine which affects the binding domain of apoprotein B.

In some series this mutation has been found in 2% of individuals with clinical FH. The mutation has also been found in individuals with either normal or only modest hypercholesterolaemia. Much still needs to be learned about this disease, particularly why some individuals develop a florid clinical picture with premature CHD whilst others remain asymptomatic.

Presumably much useful information will result from studies of carriers of this mutation with normal cholesterol levels in terms of other controlling factors for plasma cholesterol levels. Clinically those individuals with FDB resembling FH patients are treated in the same way and their response to drug therapy is similar.

FAMILIAL COMBINED HYPERLIPIDAEMIA (FCH)

Familial combined hyperlipidaemia is a well recognized clinical entity. It is more common than FH, with a frequency of approximately 0.5%, but as yet the genetics of the disorder and their interaction with environmental factors remain to be resolved. It is likely that the clinical syndrome represents a heterogeneous group of genetic abnormalities interacting with different environmental and other genetic factors.

Inheritance

FCH was first described in 1973, following a study of 500 myocardial infarction survivors and their families in Seattle, USA (Goldstein *et al.*, 1973). Of these patients (myocardial infarction < 55 years) 11% were identified as coming from families in which multiple lipoprotein abnormalities were found. Roughly a third of the affected family members had isolated hypercholesterolaemia, a third had mixed lipaemia and a third had isolated hypertriglyceridaemia.

Figure 5.3
Typical pedigree of family with familial combined hyperlipidaemia. MI = myocardial infarction. Solid black = hypercholesterol-aemia; shaded = hypertriglycerid-aemia. Source: Bierman, E.L. (1989) *Lipid Rev.* **3**, 81.

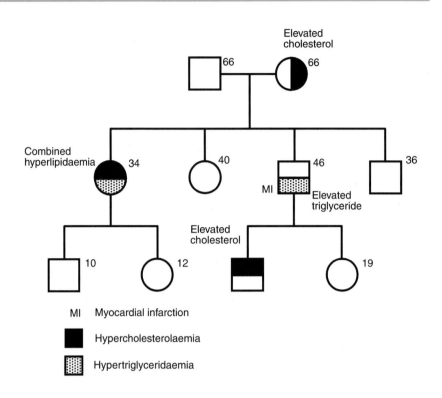

The original interpretation of the family studies was that the condition was inherited as an autosomal dominant. This has been questioned and others have suggested a polygenic inheritance. Until the genetic defects are determined, the exact inheritance will remain an open question. A typical FCH pedigree is shown in Figure 5.3.

Pathophysiology
A consistent finding in FCH is overproduction of apoprotein B-containing lipoproteins by the liver. The resulting lipid phenotype depends on the efficacy or otherwise of the catabolic pathways. It is of interest that individuals heterozygous for familial lipoprotein lipase deficiency develop a similar lipoprotein profile to FCH.

Obesity and insulin resistance appear to be commoner in FCH and undoubtedly this will contribute to the variable phenotypic expression with hypertriglyceridaemia, low HDL cholesterol, increased IDL and the presence of small, dense LDL. Apoprotein B concentrations are increased in FCH with often a decrease in LDL cholesterol : apoB ratio, indicating an increased number of lipoprotein particles.

An association has been described between the presence of coronary atherosclerosis and what was termed hyperapobetalipoproteinaemia, i.e. increased apoprotein B but normal cholesterol levels in LDL. Frequently these individuals were also hypertriglyceridaemic. The question arises as to whether these individuals should be considered as FCH.

Clinical features

There are no typical clinical stigmata to help in the diagnosis of FCH. Tendon xanthomata do not occur. Although affected individuals may have corneal arcus and xanthelasma, these signs are not specific and may be seen in individuals without lipid abnormalities.

The diagnosis is often presumptive in a patient with mixed lipaemia and CHD or a strong family history of CHD. A low HDL cholesterol and increased apoprotein B concentration (if available) are usually present. The primary care physician is well placed to perform family screening. This forms the crux of the diagnosis: the identification of family members (roughly 50%) with multiple lipoprotein phenotypes. Unlike FH, the disease is not usually expressed until late teens or early twenties.

The main reason for making the effort at diagnosis is the high CHD risk of affected individuals, including those with isolated hypertriglyceridaemia. The high risk warrants effective therapy for primary as well as secondary CHD prevention. Dietary measures are generally insufficient and drug therapy is often required, sometimes with combination therapy.

Interestingly the lipid phenotype may change with therapy. For instance, an obese individual with mixed lipaemia (type IIb) who responds well to diet may revert to type IIa phenotype. Conversely, an individual treated with a resin drug (which may exacerbate hypertriglyceridaemia) may change from a type IIa to a IIb phenotype.

COMMON POLYGENIC HYPERCHOLESTEROLAEMIA

This diagnosis fits the majority of patients with hypercholesterolaemia. It is really a diagnosis made after exclusion of secondary causes and the monogenic primary disorders. Polygenic hypercholesterolaemia reflects the interaction of multiple genes with environmental factors such as diet. It represents a heterogeneous group of disorders and classification will depend on the fruits of further research to pinpoint the major genetic susceptibility genes. The frequency of this disorder will vary between countries, principally as a result of different dietary intakes of saturated fat and cholesterol. It contributes significantly to differing mean cholesterol concentrations and CHD prevalence observed between countries.

Several common polymorphisms in different gene loci have been shown to determine differences in plasma cholesterol between individuals – the most studied being apoprotein E, apoprotein B and the LDL receptor gene. For instance, individuals carrying the apoprotein E_2 allele will on average have lower plasma cholesterol concentrations (roughly 10%) than individuals with other E alleles. Individuals with one or more E_4 alleles will on average have cholesterol concentrations 10% higher (Davignon *et al.*, 1988).

A particular polymorphism of the apoprotein B gene (identified by the presence of a cutting site with the enzyme XbaI) has been shown to be associated with increased plasma cholesterol (Humphries *et al.*, 1992). This effect is only modest (3–8%), but it is clear that the effect may be marked if this genetic polymorphism is present in an individual with other known or as yet undescribed polymorphisms at important candidate genes.

In the myocardial infarction survivor study of Goldstein *et al.* (1973) a group of patients with hypercholesterolaemia was identified whose families showed increased cholesterol levels. The prevalence of common polygenic hypercholesterolaemia will vary depending on what cut-point is taken for cholesterol. A cut-point of 7.4 mmol/l was taken in the myocardial infarction survivors study which gave a figure of 14% for the frequency of the disorder.

Patients with polygenic hypercholesterolaemia do not develop any specific physical signs although corneal arcus and xanthelasmata may be present. The degree of therapy will depend mainly on assessment of overall CHD risk. Nutritional and life style measures are the first-line therapy for those considered to be at low to moderate risk, whilst hypolipidaemic drug therapy is reserved for those at highest risk.

PRIMARY ISOLATED HYPERTRIGLYCERIDAEMIA

The large majority of patients with hypertriglyceridaemia have a demonstrable secondary cause but in some cases the disease appears to be familial and with dominant inheritance. The metabolic abnormality appears to be an increased hepatic output of large VLDL with an increased triglyceride : apoprotein B ratio. The genetic abnormality is not yet determined. LDL and HDL cholesterol concentrations tend to be low.

The degree of hypertriglyceridaemia will depend on whether there are additional acquired or genetic factors present to accentuate overproduction or impair the catabolism of the lipoproteins. Lipoprotein lipase activity is in the normal range but often towards the lower end of normal.

The diagnosis of familial hypertriglyceridaemia is made in an individual with isolated hypertriglyceridaemia together with demonstration of a similar lipid profile in other family members. This will differentiate it from FCH where multiple lipoprotein phenotypes would be expected. Unlike lipoprotein lipase deficiency, reduction of dietary fat will not lead to rapid amelioration of the hypertriglyceridaemia.

Individuals with familial hypertriglyceridaemia have either the type IV or the type V WHO phenotype. Those with the type V phenotype may develop the clinical signs described for the chylomicronaemia syndrome and are at risk of pancreatitis. To what extent CHD risk is increased in familial hypertriglyceridaemia is uncertain. As with other hypertriglyceridaemias (apart from lipoprotein lipase deficiency) glucose intolerance is a common accompaniment and the question arises as to whether it is insulin resistance that causes the hypertriglyceridaemia or vice versa.

Treatment of familial hypertriglyceridaemia is with nutrition and lifestyle measures together with hypolipidaemia drugs. The justification for treatment is to reduce the risk of pancreatitis, particularly in those with the type V phenotype.

The drugs of choice are fibrates, nicotinic acid and fish oils. With treatment, LDL concentrations paradoxically rise, but from low levels towards the normal range. There is evidence that non-receptor mediated LDL catabolism is increased in hypertriglyceridaemic states and this is reduced when the triglycerides are reduced. LDL from hypertriglyceridaemic patients binds less well to the LDL receptor, which may explain this phenomenon. The use of drugs for moderate hypertriglyceridaemia remains controversial.

REMNANT PARTICLE DISEASE

Although rare, remnant particle disease (Type III hyperlipidaemia broad-beta disease, dysbetalipoproteinaemia) is particularly interesting as it represents an interaction between established genetic and other secondary factors (either genetic or acquired). It has provided evidence of the atherogenicity of remnant particles that is of relevance to other dyslipidaemias, such as those that accompany non-insulin-dependent diabetes mellitus and insulin resistance and renal disease. Furthermore it has become clear that apoprotein E isoforms not only form the basis of remnant particle disease but also make an impact on plasma cholesterol levels in the general population (see section above on polygenic hypercholesterolaemia, p. 111).

Laboratory findings

Patients with remnant particle disease have roughly equivalent elevations in plasma cholesterol and triglyceride. In addition there are classical findings on electrophoresis and ultracentrifugation which reflect the accumulation of the remnants of chylomicron and VLDL metabolism. Lipoprotein electrophoresis shows the characteristic broad-beta band, and following separation of VLDL by ultracentrifugation the VLDL cholesterol to total triglyceride molar ratio is increased to greater than 0.6. These investigations can be performed in specialist centres but they are not necessary for effective therapy as long as the clinical syndrome is recognized, together with its importance as a cause of premature atherosclerosis affecting coronary, peripheral and cerebral vessels.

Figure 5.4

Common genetic polymorphisms of apoprotein E.

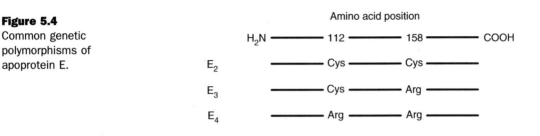

Pathophysiology

Over 90% of individuals with remnant particle disease are homozygous for the apoprotein E_2 isoform. There are three common genetically determined isoforms of apoprotein E, as shown in Figure 5.4. Approximately two-thirds of individuals are homozygous for E_3 (the normal allele) whilst E_2 homozygosity is found in approximately 1% of the population. In apoprotein E_2, cysteine substitutes for arginine at position 158. As a result, the ability of the apoprotein to bind to the LDL receptor (apoprotein B,E) is dramatically reduced.

Apoprotein E_2 homozygosity is relatively common (1 : 100) but remnant particle disease is rare, affecting between 1 : 5000 to 1 : 10 000 adults. It is clear, therefore, that further abnormalities are necessary to 'stress' the system so that dyslipidaemia develops. The other factors may be genetic, such as FCH, familial hypertriglyceridaemia and FH, or environmental, such as obesity, diabetes mellitus or hypothyroidism. With the increasing availability of isoelectric focusing or PCR techniques, the identification of E_2 homozygosity has become the confirmatory test. Very rarely remnant disease is associated with rare variants of apoprotein E or its complete absence.

As an aside, it is important to remember that possession of the apoprotein E_4 isoform has been shown to be a risk factor for the development of Alzheimer's disease. Therefore when requesting apoprotein E isoforms the request should be: is the apoprotein E isoform compatible with remnant disease? The laboratory should report along similar lines, i.e. compatible or not compatible with remnant disease, rather than reporting the actual E isoforms.

Clinical features

Remnant disease is associated with striking clinical stigmata (Plate 5). Yellow/orange streaking of the palmar creases together with soft tissue xanthomata either side of the crease are called palmar xanthoma. In addition, tuberous xanthomata resembling cauliflower florets are often present at the elbows and knees. Sometimes tuberous xanthomata are surrounded by satellite lesions resembling eruptive xanthomata, these are known as tubero-eruptive xanthomata. With coexistent FH, tendon xanthomata may be present.

Premature and extensive atherosclerosis is the most important clinical feature of remnant disease. In one series about 30% had premature CHD and a similar proportion had peripheral vascular disease. Occasionally, if the triglycerides are grossly elevated with hyperchylomicronaemia, pancreatitis may occur.

Remnant disease is generally expressed in early adult life and the diagnosis is easy when the classical stigmata are present. The contributing secondary factors need to be identified and treated appropriately if present. Treatment is with diet and hypolipidaemic drugs. The response to diet can be encouraging, particularly in the obese. If drugs are required then excellent responses are observed with either the fibrates or the HMG-CoA reductase inhibitors.

LIPOPROTEIN LIPASE DEFICIENCY (FAMILIAL CHYLOMICRONAEMIA SYNDROME)

This very rare condition is informative in that it emphasizes the importance of the enzyme, lipoprotein lipase, in lipid metabolism and the role of apoprotein C-II as the essential activator of the enzyme. It can produce severe symptoms which may go undiagnosed.

Inheritance

Absence (or virtual absence) of lipoprotein lipase activity is inherited as a recessive and presents in childhood or early adult life. In some individuals no enzyme protein is detectable; in others the enzyme protein is defective and its catalytic activity markedly reduced. In many patients the genetic defect can be identified at the molecular level. Other individuals possess normal lipoprotein lipase activity but lack apoprotein C-II, which is necessary for activation of the enzyme.

Pathophysiology

Loss of lipoprotein lipase activity results in massive accumulation of chylomicrons so that plasma triglyceride concentrations may be as high as 50–100 mmol/l. VLDL concentrations are normal and LDL and HDL concentrations decreased. Absence of lipoprotein lipase or C-II deficiency can be demonstrated in specialist centres. The diagnosis can be predicted from the massive hypertriglyceridaemia, the presence of chylomicrons in fasting plasma and the absence of secondary causes such as uncontrolled diabetes mellitus or type I glycogen storage disease, which can produce high triglyceride concentrations in children. If fasting plasma is refrigerated overnight, the characteristic cream layer is observed (Plate 6).

Clinical features

Clinically the condition presents with recurrent attacks of abdominal pain and sometimes frank pancreatitis. The risk of CHD is not increased. In addition eruptive xanthomata (Plate 7) may appear over elbows, knees and buttocks. Hepatosplenomegaly can occur, due to the accumulation of lipid-laden macrophages, and lipaemia retinalis may be observed.

An important practical point that has led to management difficulties in our experience is that massive hypertriglyceridaemia can lead to interference with amylase assays, producing falsely low levels. As a result the diagnosis of pancreatitis may be missed.

Drug therapy is ineffective in this condition and diet is the cornerstone of therapy to prevent recurrent attacks of abdominal pain. A low total fat diet is required with triglyceride intake of less than 50 g/day. This will reduce chylomicron formation and maintain plasma triglyceride levels at a level (< 20 mmol/l) unlikely to precipitate pancreatitis. No more than 20 g of fat should be eaten at any one meal. The diet may be supplemented with medium-chain triglycerides, which are absorbed directly into the portal system, but these may not be well tolerated. Other secondary causes of hypertriglyceridaemia should be avoided – including alcohol and drugs, which can increase VLDL. Patients need very careful monitoring during pregnancy.

HDL ABNORMALITIES

Occasionally hypercholesterolaemia is found to be due to a high HDL cholesterol concentration (hyperalphalipoproteinaemia). This finding represents a heterogeneous entity, with some individuals showing autosomal dominant inheritance on family screening. The diagnosis is made if HDL cholesterol (and apoprotein A-I if available) is above the 90th centile for the population in the absence of other factors known to affect HDL. The genetic basis remains to be determined. Longevity has been reported with this condition. Obviously when this diagnosis is made the patient should be reassured.

Hypoalphalipoproteinaemia is diagnosed when HDL cholesterol is below the 10th centile for the population, with normal plasma cholesterol and triglyceride concentrations. The metabolic basis for the low HDL is decreased production of apoprotein A-I. This condition is associated with increased CHD risk.

The low HDL is relatively resistant to treatment with lifestyle measures or drugs, such as fibrates, which normally increase HDL. In this situation it is our practice to lower the LDL cholesterol with drugs to 2 mmol/l in those with CHD.

Risk assessment

We have seen how the risk factor concept evolved in the 1960s from the evaluation of long-term epidemiological studies in which individual characteristics were related to the subsequent incidence of CHD. More than 280 such associations have been published, ranging from the established risk factors of dyslipidaemia, hypertension and smoking to less plausible characteristics including snoring, the speed of beard growth and even lack of attendance at church. (In the field of infectious disease, the possession of the LP 'Judy Garland – Live at the Carnegie Hall' is associated with AIDS but no one would suggest a causative role.)

The process of attributing a causative effect to an association must therefore be governed by guideline criteria:

- The association must be strong and consistent in different studies and populations.
- The association should be independent, graded and continuous – the incidence of the disease relating to levels of the risk factor.
- Prospective studies should establish an appropriate temporal sequence (the factor should precede the disease).
- The association should be plausible in terms of biological studies, clinical observations and controlled trials of risk factor reduction.

Using these criteria, the major risk factors for CHD all qualify as causal risks for CHD. Their influence on risk is powerful, common and amenable to prevention or treatment.

Summary of the evidence for a positive relationship between lipids and CHD

CHOLESTEROL

- **Epidemiological evidence:**
  - between countries – Seven Countries Study;
  - migration – Ni Hon San;
  - within countries – MRFIT, Framingham, BRHS.

  The relationship between CHD and cholesterol levels is continuous, graded and curvilinear. The risk becomes increasingly steep as cholesterol concentration increases.
- **Clinical studies**

  Genetic disorders such as familial hypercholesterolaemia relate high cholesterol levels to premature CHD.
- **Experimental studies**

  Animal studies link hypercholesterolaemia with premature atherosclerosis and studies on the mechanisms of atherogenesis *in vitro* confirm the causative link with LDL.
- **Clinical trial evidence**

  Cholesterol lowering by diet or drug therapy is associated with a reduction in CHD.

HDL CHOLESTEROL

That HDL is also a powerful and independent predictor of CHD is shown in Framingham data (Table 6.1).

The relationship is inverse, low levels of HDL being associated with increased risk of CHD. This relationship is particularly important in women. Low levels of HDL often reflect obesity, smoking, lack of exercise or impaired glucose tolerance but genetic influences may also be responsible. No prospective trial has been targeted specifically at HDL to determine whether CHD events can be reduced by increasing HDL. However, in some

Table 6.1
HDL cholesterol and CHD rates (Framingham)

HDL mmol/l	CHD rate/1000 population
<0.65	177
0.65–1.38	103
1.40–1.64	54
1.65–1.90	25

drug trials (e.g. the Helsinki Heart Study) a rise in HDL appears to contribute to CHD risk reduction.

Levels < 0.9 mmol/l in a man and < 1.1 mmol/l in a woman are negative risk factors; levels > 1.5 mmol/l in a man and > 1.7 mmol/l in a woman appear to be protective.

TRIGLYCERIDES

Evidence for triglycerides as an independent risk factor is often flawed and lacks consistency. Studies incorporating triglyceride measurement are subject to its greater measurement variability compared with other lipids due to both laboratory factors and greater short-term biological variation. The association may in fact depend on coexisting risk factors.

HDL shows a strong inverse correlation with triglycerides and studies that control for HDL usually find no independent association for triglycerides. Triglyceride levels above 1.7 mmol/l may also indicate the presence of more atherogenic subclasses of LDL (see p.18). Important associations have been described between triglycerides and factor VII and plasminogen activator inhibitor I (PAI-1).

A subgroup has emerged from observational studies (Framingham and the PROspective CArdiovascular Münster Study – PROCAM) where individuals with high triglyceride levels in the presence of low HDL seem to be at increased CHD risk. In PROCAM, 27 of 73 myocardial infarctions

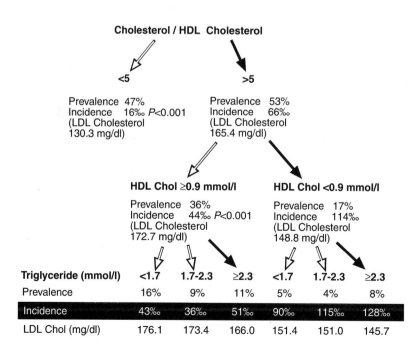

Figure 6.1
Dyslipidaemia and risk of CHD, from PROCAM (Prospective Cardiovascular Münster Study). Source: Assmann, G. *et al.* (1991), *Am. J. Cardiol.* **68** 30A–34A.
‰ = incidence per 1000

Cholesterol / HDL Cholesterol

<5

Prevalence 47%
Incidence 16‰ *P*<0.001
(LDL Cholesterol
130.3 mg/dl)

>5

Prevalence 53%
Incidence 66‰
(LDL Cholesterol
165.4 mg/dl)

HDL Chol ≥0.9 mmol/l

Prevalence 36%
Incidence 44‰ *P*<0.001
(LDL Cholesterol
172.7 mg/dl)

HDL Chol <0.9 mmol/l

Prevalence 17%
Incidence 114‰
(LDL Cholesterol
148.8 mg/dl)

Triglyceride (mmol/l)	<1.7	1.7-2.3	≥2.3	<1.7	1.7-2.3	≥2.3
Prevalence	16%	9%	11%	5%	4%	8%
Incidence	43‰	36‰	51‰	90‰	115‰	128‰
LDL Chol (mg/dl)	176.1	173.4	166.0	151.4	151.0	145.7

occurred in 8% of the subjects in whom the ratio of serum cholesterol to HDL cholesterol was > 5, the level of HDL was low and triglyceride was elevated (Figure 6.1). This pattern of raised triglyceride and low HDL with smaller denser LDL has become known as 'the atherogenic profile' and is commonly found in diabetic patients.

Again, there are no intervention trials specifically targeting triglyceride reduction but subanalysis of the Helsinki Heart Study suggested gemfibrozil exerted its most beneficial effect on the group with moderate hyper-triglyceridaemia and LDL : HDL ratio > 5.

Considering the greater accuracy in measurement and predictive capacity of serum cholesterol and HDL, the usefulness of triglyceride levels may be as a marker for atherogenic patterns. Estimation of triglyceride levels remains useful also for LDL calculation and for those patients whose hypertriglyceridaemia exposes them to the risk of pancreatitis.

Risk factors for CHD

From the intervention viewpoint it is useful to list risk factors according to their potential for modification (Table 6.2).

Clearly the 'western' diet with its high positive energy balance, high content of saturated fats and dietary cholesterol and high sugar, sodium and alcohol intake is also a necessary precondition for a high population rate of CHD. Diet mediates its effects through several risk factors and is discussed in Chapter 8.

Risk factors seldom occur in isolation and tend to 'cluster' in individuals. For example, individuals with low HDL and high triglyceride may also have

Table 6.2
Risk factors for CHD

Non-modifiable	Modifiable
Age	HYPERLIPIDAEMIA
Sex	(especially high LDL, low
Family history of CHD	HDL and high TG/low HDL)
Personal history of CHD,	HYPERTENSION
peripheral or cerebrovascular	SMOKING
disease	Diabetes mellitus and impaired
	glucose tolerance
	Obesity
	Lack of exercise
	Coagulation factors
	Psychosocial factors

truncal obesity, hypertension and impaired glucose tolerance with hyper-insulinaemia – the so-called insulin resistance syndrome (p. 131). Even without glucose intolerance, patients with hypertension tend to have above-average cholesterol levels.

When risk factors coincide, it is well known that their effect is often multiplicative rather than additive. Using MRFIT data, a smoker with a cholesterol level > 6.2 mmol/l and with a diastolic blood pressure > 90 mm Hg has, over a six-year period, a 14-fold greater CHD mortality than a non-smoker with cholesterol and diastolic pressure below these limits.

For several risk factors there are no clearly defined threshold levels at which increased risk begins. This is particularly the case for serum cholesterol and blood pressure, and dichotomous thinking that suggests an individual either has or does not have one of these risk factors is inappropriate. Whilst an individual may be either of male sex or not, the contribution from risk factors that are distributed across a range will be a question of degree.

It is important to assess the global risk of CHD for an individual to predict a prognosis, choose intervention options if necessary and select therapeutic targets. Cholesterol levels must be interpreted and treated only in the light of their clinical and biochemical context, i.e. on the basis of the global risk. Global risk is increased by:

- the presence of pre-existing atherosclerosis (CHD, PVD, etc.);
- the presence of two or more risk factors;
- the presence of a single, severe risk factor.

Non-modifiable risk factors

AGE

The absolute risk of CHD mortality and morbidity increases sharply with age. Framingham data demonstrate that a 60-year-old man with no risk factors has the same CHD mortality risk as a 45-year-old smoker with hypertension and hypercholesterolaemia.

Coronary atherosclerosis is present in 60% of autopsies on individuals aged over 65. This means that it is absent in 40% and that CHD should not be considered an inevitable consequence of ageing. That only 20% of the over 65s have CHD symptoms indicates a significant degree of asymptomatic disease in this age group.

Despite inadequate data, it seems that the classical CHD risk factors still operate in the elderly, albeit at reduced relative risk. Observational studies atios

Age	Sex ratio CHD death Male : Fenale
35–44	6.8
45–54	5.3
55–64	3.3
65–74	2.3
75+	1.6

indicate that lowering blood pressure (p. 125) and stopping smoking are beneficial but the overall risk–benefit balance of cholesterol lowering by medication has not been evaluated.

SEX

The male preponderance of CHD mortality around the world is remarkably consistent with a male : female sex ratio of between 3 and 4 (40 and 69 years) (Figure 2.5). This is all the more remarkable when one considers the variation between countries with their very different lifestyles and CHD rates. The implication is that an intrinsic gender-mediated factor is active and much speculation has centred around oestrogen. Oophorectomy in the pre-menopause is associated with a seven-fold increased risk of CHD.

The ratio decreases with age but does not disappear even in old age and this is shown in UK data (Table 6.3).

Although after the menopause the rate of CHD increase rises to equal that of men, women appear to lag 10 years behind men in the presentation of CHD and this continues to 75+ .

Examining the other risk factors, women tend to have higher cholesterol levels (Figure 2.10), blood pressure and fibrinogen levels, and are more obese and have more diabetes than men. Favourable factors include higher HDL levels (throughout life), lower triglyceride levels and less central obesity. Diabetes is the only common condition that equalizes the difference between the sexes. The protective effect of oestrogens is considered later.

FAMILY HISTORY

It is the everyday experience of clinicians that CHD is seen to cluster in some families. Family history reflects the dual influences of genetic factors and shared family environment, particularly dietary and social habits. It has proved difficult to differentiate the relative contributions of genetic and environmental factors not least because of the complex interaction of other risk factors that also have hereditary and environmental components. At an individual level, there is great variation in susceptibility to a risk factor and again both genetic and environmental factors must be active.

Framingham data shows that siblings of a brother with CHD have more than double the risk of a CHD event themselves, even after controlling for cholesterol, hypertension and smoking. A history of CHD in parents is associated with a 30% increased risk. A family history of CHD is thus established as an independent risk factor.

Recently there has been interest in the possibility that intra-uterine and perinatal experiences may exert a programming effect on the future handling of risk factors and hence provide an alternative explanation to variations in susceptibility.

Clear contributions are made by family history in the assessment of patients with genetic hyperlipidaemias, such as FH with its pattern of autosomal dominant inheritance.

When taking a family history, the interviewer needs to ascertain:

- the age of onset of disease in the affected relatives (especially if < 55 years);
- the degree of closeness of the affected relatives:
  - 1° – parents and siblings;
  - 2° – uncles, aunts, grandparents;
- the number and proportion of affected relatives;
- whether the affected relatives had other risk factors (e.g. smoking or hypertension).

A PERSONAL HISTORY OF CHD

Patients with a history of CHD are at increased risk of further events. For example, Pekkanen showed in 1990 that over a 10-year period the risk of dying from CHD was increased more than 20 times in men with previous myocardial infarction. Although the historical fact of a personal history of CHD is non-modifiable, the same risk factors associated with the initial development of CHD govern the likelihood of recurrence. The Stanford Coronary Risk Intervention Project (SCRIP) in 1994 showed that patients with CHD who made substantial improvements in their risk profiles decreased the rate of progression of their coronary atheorsclerosis and reduced hospital admissions for cardiac events. The strength of the secondary prevention trials highlights such high risk patients as priorities for intervention.

Non-lipid modifiable risk factors

HYPERTENSION

Hypertension is established as one of the major independent risk factors for CHD and satisfies the criteria suggesting a causal relationship. The major causes of death attributable to hypertension are cerebrovascular disease (stroke) and CHD and the relative incidence of these varies around the world according to the impact of other risk factors. The consequences of hypertension are:

- stroke
  - embolic, thrombotic, haemorrhagic
  - multi-infarct dementia
- coronary heart disease
- left ventricular hypertrophy
- heart failure
- renal vascular disease
- peripheral vascular disease (including aortic dissection).

There is a continuous, graded, near linear relationship between both systolic and diastolic blood pressure and CHD and stroke. This is illustrated in Figure 6.2, the size of the squares being proportional to the number of events and the vertical lines representing 95% confidence intervals.

It can be seen that the majority of strokes and CHD events occur in 'normotensives' (i.e. individuals whose blood pressure levels would not normally warrant treatment). We have seen the same phenomenon with cholesterol (Figure 4.2) and interaction with other risk factors is responsible. Lipid risk factors coexist in the hypertensive individual more often than by chance even when confounding variables such as obesity, drug side effects and alcohol consumption are taken into account. Nutritional influences, genetic factors and the insulin resistance syndrome may provide unifying explanations for the relationship.

The definition of hypertension is consequently much debated but remains arbitrary due to the continuous and graded relationship of blood pressure to cardiovascular risk. There is no point at which blood pressure is 'safe' or suddenly becomes 'dangerous'. The WHO definition of > 160/95, whilst taking into account the point at which the attributable risk becomes really significant, does not reflect the information arising from the treatment trials in elderly hypertensives (p. 154) where a reading $\geq$ 160/90 predicts benefit from treatment.

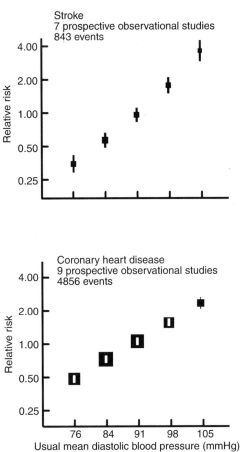

Figure 6.2

Risk of stroke and coronary heart disease associated with hypertension. Source: MacMahon *et al.* (1990) *Lancet* **335**, 765–774

From middle age onwards, systolic blood pressure is a greater predictor of CHD events than diastolic blood pressure. Systolic pressure tends to rise throughout life but diastolic pressure peaks at about 60 years and then declines (Figure 6.3). This rise is not observed in primitive societies and it cannot therefore be viewed as part of normal ageing.

The risks of blood pressure are much higher once hypertension has induced target organ damage. Left ventricular hypertrophy (LVH) is easily recognized on an ECG and is a powerful predictor of CHD events, carrying a poor prognosis if untreated. The discovery of target organ damage or the presence of other severe CHD risk factors should invoke a lower threshold for anti-hypertensive intervention and a more stringent target level.

Clinical trials of blood pressure lowering offer convincing evidence of reduction in strokes and heart failure but reduction in CHD is more modest than predicted. The interaction of other risk factors partly explains the discrepancy. For example, in the Gothenburg hypertension trial, reduced rates of CHD were largely confined to those in whom both blood pressure

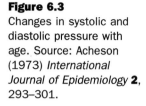

Figure 6.3
Changes in systolic and diastolic pressure with age. Source: Acheson (1973) *International Journal of Epidemiology* **2**, 293–301.

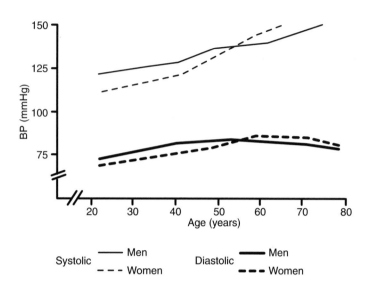

and cholesterol were reduced. Certain anti-hypertensives adversely modify lipid profiles and this is further discussed in Chapter 11.

SMOKING

The tobacco plant, *Nicotiana tabacum*, is indigenous to America and came to Europe following Christopher Columbus's voyages of exploration. For hundreds of years, North American Indians had either smoked or chewed leaves for narcotic, medicinal, religious or social purposes. Sir Walter Raleigh introduced tobacco to Britain during Elizabeth I's reign and almost immediately her government imposed a tobacco tax of two pence in the pound, recognizing an early potential for revenue generation. In 1604 James I described tobacco as 'hateful to the nose, harmful to the brain and dangerous to the lungs'. Duty had by now risen to six shillings and eight pence in the pound.

Over the next three centuries, tobacco was smoked in pipes, chewed or taken as snuff. In the early nineteenth century the first cigars were made but the development of the cigarette in the latter half of the same century provided the springboard for the huge world-wide growth in smoking behaviour. At first cigarettes were crude and hand rolled but manufacturing processes improved and the first cigarette factory in England opened in London in 1856.

Cigarette smoking dramatically increased amongst men in the UK, North America and western Europe in the decade before the first world war and rates in women soon began to increase as well. Smoking prevalence for men in the UK peaked just after the second world War (65% in 1948) but the peak for women was in the 1970s (50%). Over the last 10 years rates have dropped significantly and 28% of men and 26% of women smoked in 1994. These figures disguise high rates in certain subgroups – for example, 38% of young women aged 20–24 years. Smoking behaviour in different socio-economic groups has polarized since 1960, when there was an even spread, and now 18% of social class I males smoke compared with 39% of social class V. Fewer than 5% of British GPs now smoke. There are, however, still 14 million smokers in the UK.

World tobacco consumption is 1.9 kg/person over 15 and this figure is remarkably stable. Developed countries have cut consumption by 17% this decade and for the total consumption figure to be stable this means that developing countries have shown a corresponding increase. China now smokes 30% of world cigarettes and can expect mounting mortality from smoking-related diseases.

World-wide, the effects of smoking are estimated to kill 3 million people per year. This contrasts with 0.2 million in 1950 and projections for 2025 of 10 million. In the UK up to 150 000 deaths per year (one-sixth of the total), one-third of cancer deaths and one-quarter of CHD deaths are attributable to smoking. Thus, smoking represents the most important preventable cause of death in the developed world.

Shortly after establishing the relationship between smoking and lung cancer, Doll and Hill in 1951 set up the British Doctors Study. The 40-year follow-up is now available on the 34 439 British male doctors and it is clear that half of all regular smokers are eventually killed by their habit. Of the excess deaths in the smoking group, 31% succumbed to CHD and 21% to other cardiovascular diseases, including stroke.

Consequences of cigarette smoking
The consequences of cigarette smoking are:

- reduced lifespan (by 4.6 years in men who smoke 20/day from age 25)
- coronary heart disease
- peripheral vascular disease, aneurysm
- CVA (particularly in women using oral contraception)
- venous thrombosis
- cardiac arrhythmias
- peri-operative mortality increase
- cancer of lung, larynx, oesophagus, mouth, tongue, bladder, kidney, pancreas and cervix
- chronic obstructive airways disease
- peptic ulcer
- low birthweight infants, premature birth, miscarriage
- Crohn's disease
- osteoporosis

- passive smoking effects – asthma in infants, lung cancer
- economic costs.

Amongst cigarette smokers, risk is increased by the number of cigarettes smoked, the amount of inhalation, the age of starting, the number of years of smoking and the tar yield of the preferred cigarette. Increasing numbers of cigarettes smoked increases mortality in a near linear fashion (Figure 6.4).

Attempts have been made over the last 30 years to reduce the emission levels of tar, carbon monoxide and nicotine from cigarettes. Filters are used by 92% of men and 97% of women, and low tar cigarettes (5–15 mg per cigarette) are associated with slightly reduced mortality. The tar content of European cigarettes is restricted by the European Union to 12 mg/cigarette from 1997 in contrast to export brands. For example, Chesterfield cigarettes in the Philippines have a tar content of 31 mg. There is some evidence, unfortunately, that when switching to lower-tar brands the smoker adjusts by increasing consumption.

Primary pipe or cigar smokers have almost the risk of non-smokers but those who switch from cigarette smoking appear to receive little benefit.

Lung cancer has been confirmed as a hazard of passive smoking. In a survey of 10 epidemiological studies, nine studies found increased rates of CHD in passive smokers but statistical significance was not reached.

Mechanisms of damage

Cigarette smoke contains 3000–4000 different components and each puff contains 10^{13} free radicals. Studies in rats have demonstrated endothelial cell changes as a result of injury, and enhanced deposition of fibrinogen and

Figure 6.4
CHD mortality in male British doctors by age and smoking habit. Source: Doll and Peto (1976)

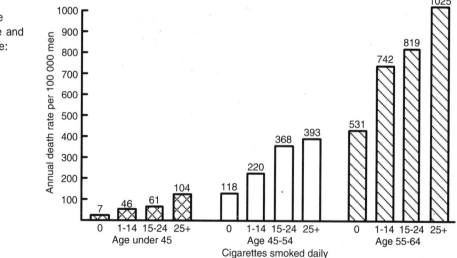

lipids contributes to atherogenesis. Fibrinogen levels and platelet aggregation are increased and this leads to increased blood coagulability and viscosity. Smoking appears to reduce HDL and increase triglycerides. By sympatho-adrenal stimulation, nicotine reduces coronary blood flow – most markedly in areas already compromised by ischaemic damage – and this may precipitate arrhythmias or angina, potentially resulting in the observed increased risk of sudden death among smokers.

Smoking in young people

By 15, more than one in four English schoolchildren smoke cigarettes regularly (Figure 6.5). In 1990, 28% of male and 32% of female 16–19 year-olds smoked regularly. Children who smoke are influenced by the habits of their peers, parents and particularly their siblings and there is good evidence that they smoke the most heavily advertised brands. In 1994, the UK government was estimated to receive £108 million in tax from cigarettes sold illegally to children under 16. Total revenue in this year from tobacco taxation was £8463 million and the taxation rate has now risen to 80p in the pound.

Stopping smoking

There is little doubt that stopping smoking can reduce CHD risk. The Oslo study (p. 57) provides convincing evidence, as does a study from Sweden which showed 85% survival at five years in a group of non-smoking female MI survivors compared with 73% survival in the group who continued to smoke. Where there is doubt is how quickly the benefits of cessation are

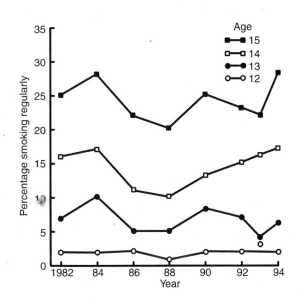

Figure 6.5
Percentage of English schoolchildren (by age) smoking regularly. Source: *OPCS Survey of smoking among secondary schoolchildren, 1982–1994.*

achieved. Here surveys vary: in the BRHS the risk for heavy smokers remained increased for more than 20 years after stopping, whereas Framingham data suggests a much swifter effect. Changes in coagulation and rheological (flow) factors are improved within 48 hours of cessation and it may be that the benefits are more rapid than was previously thought.

DIABETES AND IMPAIRED GLUCOSE TOLERANCE

Whilst their atherosclerotic lesions are similar, the atheroma of diabetics is more extensive and diffuse compared with non-diabetics. Three-quarters of diabetics die from large vessel (macrovascular) disease and a half from CHD, with significant contributions from cerebrovascular disease and peripheral vascular disease. In the Joslin clinic in Boston, CHD mortality amongst insulin-dependent diabetics was 35% by the age of 55. The presence of diabetic renal disease with microalbuminuria or proteinuria greatly enhances the risk of CHD.

Diabetic women have a strikingly higher relative risk of CHD than men (the relative risk of CHD in Framingham diabetics was 2.4 for men and 5.1 for women). This completely eradicates the sex advantage that premenopausal women normally hold.

The increased CHD risk is probably due to the effect of conventional risk factors, which are exaggerated in diabetes and exert greater effect. Whatever the combination of other risk factors, the diabetic fares worse than the non-diabetic.

Major lipid abnormalities are more common in non-insulin-dependent diabetes mellitus (NIDDM), the commonest lipid abnormality being hypertriglyceridaemia with reduced HDL. Total cholesterol tends to be unaltered but there is more small dense atherogenic LDL3 with its increased susceptibility to oxidation.

Impaired glucose tolerance (glucose intolerance)

This term has replaced the old 'borderline' or 'chemical' diabetes and is defined as a fasting glucose of less than 7.8 mmol/l and and a level of between 7.8 and 11.1 mmol/l two hours after a 75 g glucose load. It is more common than diabetes, with a prevalence in the UK of 17% (40–65 years) and 11% in the United States (20–74 years). Whilst individuals are not at risk from microvascular complications such as retinopathy, the significance lies in a doubling of the CHD rate as shown in Whitehall data. Over 10 years about 15% become diabetics but most remain with continuing impairment. The pathogenesis is controversial – whether the condition is one of insulin deficiency or resistance.

Insulin resistance

In many populations the combination of low HDL and high triglycerides has been found in those at high risk of CHD. The associated findings of high blood glucose and high insulin levels suggest a relative insensitivity of the tissues to insulin (insulin resistance) and more insulin is required to maintain normoglycaemia. NIDDM is a late stage where increasing hyperglycaemia and hyperinsulinaemia lead to beta cell failure.

In 1988 Reaven described the clustering of diabetes or impaired glucose tolerance, hyperinsulinaemia, central obesity, hypertension, low HDL and raised triglycerides as 'Syndrome X'. (This was unfortunate as the term had already been coined to describe angiographically negative patients with angina. True Syndrome X patients, however, commonly have insulin resistance and presumably should be Syndrome XX.) The syndrome has since been described as the insulin resistance syndrome and may provide a unifying theory behind the risks of hypertension, obesity, glucose intolerance, low HDL and high triglyceride and the problems of certain ethnic groups (Figure 6.6).

OBESITY

Long-term prospective studies have consistently shown that excess body fat is related to increased levels of CHD. Many of the effects of obesity,

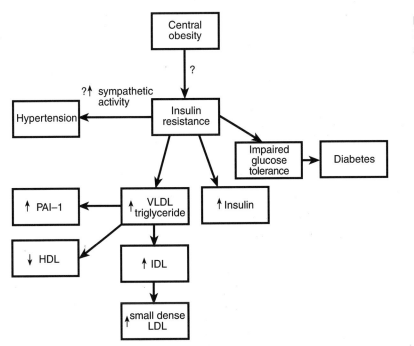

Figure 6.6
Insulin resistance syndrome.

however, are mediated through increases in other characteristics and this has led to debate concerning the independence of obesity as a risk factor.

Obesity is associated with hypertension, increased serum cholesterol and triglycerides and reduced HDL. There is also associated insulin insensitivity with increased glucose and insulin levels and increased rates of NIDDM. When studies such as the Seven Countries Study correct for these factors, obesity does not emerge as an independent risk factor, but some investigators, using the same data, have drawn different conclusions. Research from Framingham also supports independence, particularly in the under 50s and where central obesity is present. Whether obesity is an independent risk factor or merely a 'marker' for others is in practice an unnecessary distinction as it certainly represents a readily identifiable and potentially modifiable risk factor.

Fat distribution and measurement

Central, truncal or android obesity is commonly seen in men whose 'pot bellies' make them look 'apple shaped'. This pattern of obesity reflects increased intra-abdominal fat which adversely affects hepatic lipid and insulin metabolism. It is commonly seen in South Asians and is associated with the insulin resistance syndrome (pp. 41 and 121).

A thick waist and a propensity for fat deposition around the buttocks and hips, producing a 'pear shape', characterize peripheral or gynaecoid obesity. This is more common in women but the patterns are not gender specific, indeed central obesity for women confers significant CHD risk (Figure 6.7).

Obesity is measured as body mass index (BMI – Quetelet's Index) (Figure 8.1):

$$BMI \ (kg/m^2) = weight \ (kg)/height \ (m)$$

Figure 6.7
Obesity distribution: 'pear' and 'apple' body shapes.

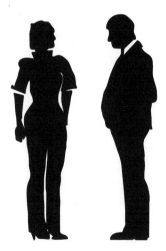

The normal range for BMI is 20–25 kg/m^2. A BMI in the range 25–30 kg/m^2 is associated with a slight increase in mortality but this climbs steeply beyond 30 kg/m^2. Whilst BMI is the commonest measure of obesity it does not always correlate well with CHD risk. For example, a short, stocky, muscular man who by his activity and fitness has a low CHD risk may have a high BMI. Measurement of fat distribution would reflect a more accurate picture.

Central obesity is best estimated by the direct ratio of waist measurement to hip measurement. The higher the ratio, the higher is the CHD risk and vice versa. Normal waist hip ratio (WHR) for a man is 0.9, for a woman 0.8.

Prevalence of obesity

The prevalence of obesity (BMI > 30 kg/m^2) in the UK doubled between 1980 and 1991 and, worryingly, continues to increase (Table 6.4).

The intense relationship with socio-economic status, especially amongst women, has already been noted (p. 40). Obesity is even more prevalent in the USA, where it exceeds 50% amongst certain female subgroups.

When secular trends are analysed, it is clear that obesity is increasing despite reductions in energy and total fat intake in the diet. Energy expenditure is declining and there are clear correlations with the numbers of cars, televisions and VCRs as well as with increasing levels of inactivity.

Consequences of obesity

The consequences of obesity are:

- coronary heart disease;
- hypertension;
- stroke;
- non-insulin-dependent diabetes mellitus (NIDDM);
- gallstones;
- increased mechanical load producing musculoskeletal disease and reduced exercise tolerance;
- fertility problems and cancer (adipose tissue contains aromatase which converts androgens to oestrogens – this contributes to infertility and sex-hormone-sensitive cancers).

BMI (kg/m^2)	1980		1994	
	Male	Female	Male	Female
25–30	33	24	43	29
> 30	6	8	13	16

Table 6.4
Increasing prevalence of obesity in UK (% total male and total female population, respectively)

LACK OF EXERCISE

Again, lack of exercise is difficult to assess as an independent risk factor because of the positive effects of exercise on other characteristics. 'Exercisers' tend to lead healthier lifestyles and of course there are no randomized controlled trials. Nevertheless, in nearly 50 epidemiological studies, none has shown higher risk of CHD in physically active men.

Using their network of past graduates, the Harvard Alumni study found the rate of myocardial infarction to be 64% higher in men who expended less than 2000 kcal/week on exercise than classmates with higher levels of activity.

Occupational exercise was neatly investigated when London double-decker-bus conductors were found to have half the incidence of CHD compared with their driver colleagues. The question of self selection arose when it was pointed out that conductors were of slimmer build than drivers and that perhaps conductors were innately healthier and able to choose more active jobs. When the trouser band width of their uniforms (a measure of central obesity?) was related to the rates of CHD, it was shown that whatever the size of the conductor – slim, normal or overweight – their rates were still half those of drivers.

Similar findings were reported in San Francisco dockworkers where those with sedentary occupations had an 80% excess risk of fatal CHD compared with the stevedores.

As the number of heavy jobs in westernized society diminishes, more exercise will need to be taken in leisure time.

Benefits of exercise

Exercise causes slight reduction in blood pressure, definite reduction in weight, improved glucose tolerance and coagulation profiles, reduced myocardial oxygen consumption and psychological and social benefits. HDL cholesterol is increased and triglycerides reduced. A study in overweight men showed that jogging an average 11.7 miles/week produced a 10.4% increase in HDL. Similarly, in middle-aged women, 2.5 hours brisk walking per week improved HDL by 27%. Vigorous exercise in post-myocardial infarction patients has been shown to reduce future events by 50%.

To be beneficial, exercise must be current and of sufficient vigour. This means the expenditure of 7.5 kcal/min and data from British civil servants suggests that vigorous sports, fast walking (> 4 mph) and cycling can all achieve this. Vigorous recreational activity (gardening, DIY), whilst beneficial, did not.

Death during recreational exercise is uncommon (4.46 deaths/100 000 men in Rhode Island) but unaccustomed strenuous exercise is to be avoided (p. 153). There is evidence from Harvard that walking 9 miles/week

Factor	MI	Angina	CHD	No CHD
Number in study	38	33	71	1350
Fibrinogen (g/l)	3.24	3.21	3.22	2.91

Table 6.5
Relationship between fibrinogen and CHD (Northwick Park Heart Study)

produces a 21% reduction in death rate. In the BRHS 40–60 minutes of walking a day again reduced risk.

Unfortunately 7/10 men and 8/10 women do not take enough exercise for a health benefit and the sedentary lifestyle is very common.

THROMBOGENIC FACTORS

Although a thrombotic component was recognized as long ago as 1912, in Herrick's description of coronary thrombosis, the role of thrombogenic factors in the development of unstable angina, myocardial infarction and sudden death was not established until the early 1980s.

The Northwick Park Heart Study (Meade, 1986) demonstrated a positive relationship between fibrinogen and CHD in a population about as strong as that for cholesterol itself (Table 6.5).

Factors VII and VIII and low fibrinolytic activity have also been associated with CHD and data from Framingham and at least four other studies confirm the findings.

Fibrinogen is not often measured in clinical practice and there is no general agreement as to which assay technique should be standard. It is a large molecule that increases blood viscosity and platelet aggregation leading to a hypercoagulable state favouring plaque thrombosis. It also has a role in atherogenesis by fibrin deposition in vessel walls.

High fibrinogen levels are most common in smokers where levels are increased by up to 10%, the rise being proportional to the number of cigarettes smoked. It is interesting that in the WHO clofibrate trial, most of the reduction in CHD was in the heavy smoking group. (Whilst clofibrate has lipid-lowering effects, it also reduces fibrinogen.)

The list of situations where fibrinogen is increased reads like a list of CHD risk factors:

- smoking
- increasing age
- obesity
- oral contraception

- diabetes/insulin resistance
- hypertension
- peripheral vascular disease
- stress
- hypercholesterolaemia
- hypertriglyceridaemia
- lack of exercise
- menopause.

Fibrinogen is decreased by:

- moderate alcohol intake
- exercise
- drugs – fibrates (especially bezafibrate, fenofibrate and ciprofibrate), nicotinic acid and increasing reports re statins.

After stopping smoking, there are differences in fibrinogen levels within two days but the return to non-smoker levels is very slow and may take 5–10 years.

PSYCHOSOCIAL FACTORS

If the relatives of a victim of CHD are asked for antecedent factors, it is inevitable that stress will figure prominently. The evidence, however, is limited, not only because stress is difficult to define and measure but also because there is great individual variation of response. A few retrospective studies have examined life events before myocardial infarction but there is no predictive link. There is a lack of studies looking at the acute crisis situation where the reaction is probably neurohumoral.

In 1959, Type A personality (competitive, aggressive, time urgent) was linked with increased CHD compared with the more passive Type B personality. In the Whitehall study of British civil servants, men of the lowest working grades had three times the CHD rates of workers in the highest grades. Although the highest grades had the lowest rates for CHD, they also included more Type A individuals and this has weakened the personality theory. Differences in traditional risk factors only partly explain the findings and it seems that an individual's position within a hierarchy is important. This is reflected in an animal model where lower order monkeys on a high fat diet develop the most atherosclerosis. Further negative influences have been identified as unemployment, job strain, lack of social support, social inequality and lower educational attainment.

Recently, Type D personality (unhappy, gloomy, prone to depression and worrying) has been shown to be a significant predictor of mortality in CHD patients. In one study, a link between a boring job and high fibrinogen levels has been established and variations in coagulation factors may in future provide the link between stress and the acute coronary event.

HOMOCYSTEINE

Homocysteine is a sulphur amino acid produced by demethylation of the essential amino acid, methionine. If plasma homocysteine concentrations are sufficiently high, urinary excretion occurs and the disulphide homocystine can be detected in the urine. It has been known for years that patients with the homozygous condition, homocystinuria (classically deficiency of the breakdown enzyme, cystathionine β-synthetase), die from premature atherosclerosis. Now more than 40 case control studies implicate raised plasma homocysteine levels as a risk factor for coronary, cerebral and peripheral atherosclerosis.

For example, the European Union Concerted Action Project's analysis of 1550 patients found that those with homocysteine levels in the top quintile (> 12 μmol/l) experienced double the risk of myocardial infarction in both men and women.

The mechanism whereby homocysteine may exert its action is not clear but experimental evidence points to its ability to damage endothelium, to affect platelet function and coagulation factors and to promote LDL oxidation. Interaction with other conventional risk factors further increases risk.

Vitamins B6, B12 and folic acid all act as co-factors in homocysteine metabolism and both folate and B12 relate inversely to homocysteine concentration. Dietary supplementation with folic acid (200–400 μg/day) reduces plasma homocysteine by about 30% and offers the potential for therapy. A large secondary prevention trial (HERMIT) will evaluate this potential and establish the practical significance of homocysteine as a major coronary risk factor.

Alcohol as a risk factor

More than sixty studies have shown that people who drink small amounts of alcohol have lower rates of CHD than those who drink heavily or not at all. Expressed graphically, this is known as the U-shaped curve. Moderate alcohol consumption appears to be cardioprotective, with a relative risk reduction of the order of 0.5–0.7 even when confounding variables are accounted for.

People who do not drink alcohol are a composite group formed of those who have never drunk alcohol ('never drinkers') and those who have had to give up alcohol because of some other health problem ('sick quitters'). At least four analyses, which included 'never drinkers', confirm the validity of the U-shaped curve (Figure 6.8).

Although higher rates of CHD do not begin to appear in men until levels of about 40 units/week are reached, all-cause mortality climbs from levels around 21 units/week and this fits closely with recommended advice. Beyond 21 units/week there are rises in cirrhosis, accidents, haemorrhagic CVA and sociopathic problems. The lowest all-cause mortality is found at 7 units/week. Under the age of 40, any alcohol consumption is associated with increased mortality because CHD rates are low and the risk of death by injury is relatively high. The CHD benefits begin to accrue in men over the age of 40 and women over 50 and continue into old age.

Alcohol produces a beneficial rise in HDL cholesterol (HDL2 and HDL3) but at moderate intake and beyond there is a concomitant rise in triglycerides and VLDL. Fibrinogen is reduced and there are beneficial influences on platelet aggregation and plasminogen activation. There is also a transient rise in blood pressure reflecting consumption over the preceding days which takes several more days of abstention to settle. Clearly chronic drinking remains an important cause of reversible hypertension. Unfortunately the beneficial effect of increased HDL is therefore offset by rises in triglycerides, VLDL and blood pressure as consumption increases.

Figure 6.8
The U-shaped curve: relative risk of acute myocardial infarction and number of drinks per week. Source: Jackson *et al*. (1991) *BMJ* **303**, 211–216.

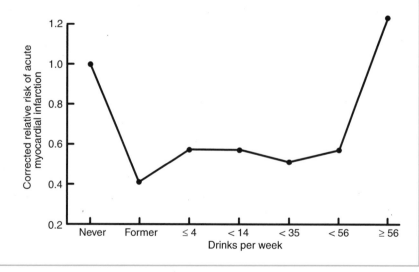

Apart from the debate regarding quantity of alcohol, there has also been debate regarding type. A recent analysis by Rimm (1996) suggests that probably all alcoholic drinks can exert cardioprotection, but prior surveys have extolled the virtues of wine and the Copenhagen City Heart Study showed increased CHD risk in spirit drinkers. Rimm is supported by data from Shanghai (1997) where moderate alcohol consumption is again associated with a reduced risk of death. In this non-Western population (where grape wine consumption, incidentally, is very low) the type of alcohol makes no difference.

Intervention priorities, action limits and targets

We have seen that it is an individual's overall risk of CHD that determines the benefit of an intervention such as cholesterol lowering and that cholesterol cannot be considered in isolation from the other risk factors. Moreover, strategies to benefit individuals at high risk need to be more stringent.

Whilst the primary prevention of CHD for a population (with public health measures and risk assessment for everyone) may be the ultimate goal, there is a logistic problem due to the large numbers of people involved. There is considerable potential in tackling secondary prevention first and every GP in the UK has at least 50 patients with CHD. The reinfarction rate following myocardial infarction is 30% and lipid lowering, smoking cessation, the use of beta blockers and modification of coagulation factors with aspirin all confer benefit. Secondary prevention trials of cholesterol lowering demonstrate reduced CHD events and lower total mortality and represent a more rapid, efficient and cost-effective mechanism for reducing the CHD burden of an affected country.

A crude initial guide for action limits for lipid level reduction can be taken as:

- cholesterol > 5.2 mmol/l
- HDL < 0.9 mmol/l
- triglyceride > 2.3 mmol/l
- LDL > 4.0 mmol/l.

Patients whose cholesterol level is less than 4.5 mmol/l or more than 8 mmol/l, where either no treatment or definite active treatment is required, pose few dilemmas. Patients with levels between 4.5 and 8 mmol/l need the application of clinical judgment to place the level of cholesterol in context with the presence, severity and number of other risk factors. Some risk factors are either present or absent (e.g. male sex) but others (e.g. choles-terol, blood pressure) vary in severity. We have seen how the interaction of several risk factors is multiplicative.

In 1993 the **British Hyperlipidaemia Association** published guidelines for the management of patients with hyperlipidaemia. All patients with hyperlipidaemia should receive dietary and lifestyle advice but the priorities and action limits for lipid-lowering drug therapy in diet-resistant patients is shown in Table 5.2c.

Placing patients with CHD, multiple risk factors and genetic disorders at high priority reflects the current state of understanding that patients at high risk benefit most from intervention. Unfortunately, many high risk patients are being denied the benefits of lipid lowering therapy. Less than 0.1% of the population in the UK receive lipid lowering drugs, a figure somewhat removed from the 2–3% of the population known to have CHD (approx-imately 50 patients per GP). One study showed that only 23% of diabetics with cholesterol levels in excess of 7.8 mmol/l were prescribed lipid-lowering medication and many hypertensives would also qualify for more active treatment.

The European Atherosclerosis Society (EAS) published guidelines for CHD prevention in 1992 and their target levels for cholesterol and LDL are shown in Table 6.6 (see also Table 5.2b). The major focus of these target levels is LDL, recognizing the fact that it is the prime determinant of CHD. This focus is common to other national and international guidelines which are now remarkably similar in their recommendations, particularly in their emphasis on overall risk assessment prior to planning treatment.

In the United States in 1993, the National Cholesterol Education Program Expert Panel on Detection, Evaluation and Treatment of High Blood Cholesterol in Adults second report was published (**ATP II**). Three levels of risk are identified:

- highest risk – patients with CHD;
- high risk – high cholesterol and multiple risk factors;
- lower risk – high cholesterol but no other risk factors.

The need for aggressive cholesterol lowering in patients at highest risk is emphasized but patients with peripheral vascular and carotid artery disease are also included. For patients with PVD or after a TIA, CHD is the major cause of death.

Similarly, aggressive cholesterol lowering is recommended for diabetics, including women. Age is added as a major risk factor, defined as > 45 years for men and > 55 years for women. Amongst the elderly, those at high risk who are otherwise in good health may benefit from treatment and HRT

Global risk	Cholesterol goal mmol/l	LDL goal mmol/l
Mild risk e.g. TC 5.2–7.8, no non-lipid risk factors	5.0–6.0	4.0–4.5
Moderate risk e.g. TC 5.2–7.8, plus 1 non-lipid risk factor or plus HDL < 1.0 (especially < 0.8)	5.0	3.5–4.0
High risk e.g. CHD/PVD or TC > 7.8 or familial syndrome or TC 5.2–7.8 plus 2 non-lipid risk factors or TC 5.2–7.8 plus 1 severe non-lipid risk factor	4.5–5.0 (?4.0–4.5 and 2.5 in secondary prevention)	3.0–3.5

Table 6.6
European Atherosclerosis Society guidelines for CHD prevention (1992): target levels for cholesterol and LDL

should be considered for post-menopausal women at risk rather than lipid-lowering drugs.

More attention is given to HDL, and HDL < 0.9 mmol/l is added as a major risk factor and > 1.6 mmol/l as a negative (protective) one. In secondary prevention, LDL target levels of < 2.6 mmol/l are advocated and the action limits and LDL targets are summarized in Table 5.2a.

In 1994 a joint European Task Force representing the European Society of Cardiology, the European Atherosclerosis Society and the European Society of Hypertension published consensus guidelines (**ESC**). Again, there is striking agreement with other guidelines with emphasis on risk stratification and aggressive intervention for those at highest risk. The ESC guidelines use coronary risk charts devised by Anderson *et al.* in 1991 from Framingham data. The estimation of the risk of future CHD events is complex as so many variables exert influence. An absolute risk of 2% per annum (or 20% per 10 years) describes the chance of CHD events in that time. The coronary risk chart allows prediction of a patient's absolute 10-year risk of a CHD event based on the risk factors of total cholesterol, age, sex, smoking habit and systolic blood pressure. Treatment is advocated if 10-year risk exceeds 20% (Figures 6.9 and 6.10).

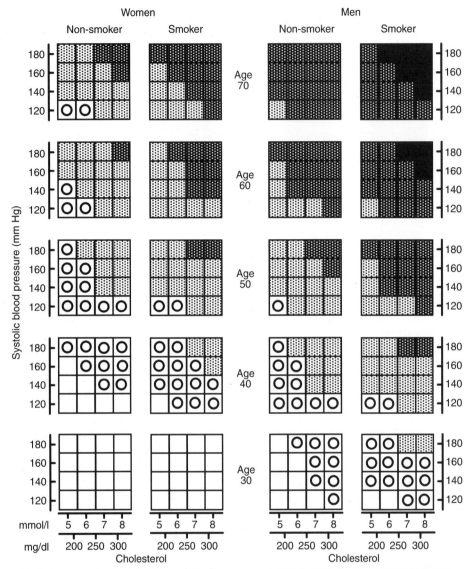

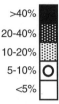

• To find a person's absolute 10-year risk of a CHD event, find the table for their sex, age and smoking status. Inside the table, find the cell nearest to their systolic blood pressure (mm Hg) and cholesterol (mmol/l or mg/dl).

• To find a person's relative risk, compare their risk category with other people of the same age. The absolute risk shown here may not apply to all populations, especially those with a low CHD incidence. Relative risk is likely to apply to most populations.

• The effect of changing cholesterol, smoking status or blood pressure can be read from the chart.

• The effect of lifetime exposure to risk factors can be seen by following the table upwards. This can be used when advising younger people

• Risk is at least one category higher in people with overt cardiovasular disease. People with diabetes, familial hyperlipidaemia or a family history of premature cardiovascular disease are also at increased risk.

• Risks are shown for exact ages, blood pressures and cholesterols. Risk increases as a person approaches the next category.

• The tables assume HDL cholesterol to be 1.0 mmol/l in men (39 mg/dl) and 1.1 mmol/l (43 mg/dl) in women. People with lower levels of HDL cholesterol and/or with triglyceride levels above 2.3 mmol/l (200 mg/dl) are at higher risk.

• Cholesterol: 1 mmol/l=38.67 mg/dl.

Figure 6.9
Coronary Risk Chart. Source: Pyörälä *et al.* (1994) Prevention of CHD in clinical practice: recommendations of the task force of the ESC, EAS and ESH. *European Heart Journal* **15** 1300–1331.

Total cardiovascular risk should be assessed first and the major components of risk identified. If 10-year CHD risk exceeds 20% or will exceed 20% if projected to age 60 more intensive advice for all risk factors will be required. Clinical vascular disease will increase the risk to more than 20% for most and to more than 40% for many.

Cholesterol level mg/dl mmol/l	General risk factor advice	Intensive physician- and dietician-directed risk advice	Drug treatment considered if diet fails	Comment
350 — ⌐ 9	→	Yes	Yes	Check fasting lipids Exclude secondary hyperlipidaemia Check family members
300 — ⌐ 8	→	Yes	Yes if CHD risk > 20%	Check fasting lipids Exclude secondary hyperlipidaemia
250 — ⌐ 7 ⌐ 6	Yes	Yes if CHD risk > 20%	Occasionally if very high risk	
200 — ⌐ 5	Yes	Yes if CHD risk > 20%		

- Diet is the cornerstone of management.
- General risk factor advice implies avoidance of tobacco, weight control, less than 30% of dietary calories as fat (of which less than 1/3rd saturated),control of hypertension and frequent leisure exercise.
- Management decisions should not be based on a single cholesterol measurement. Laboratory variation may be 0.5 mmol/l (20 mg/dl) or more.

- Raised triglycerides signal the need for fasting lipid estimations (HDL cholesterol may be low) Hypertriglyceridaemia often responds to weight and alcohol control.
- The benefits or otherwise of drug treatment in women and in the elderly are unknown

Recently in the UK Ramsey *et al.* (1996) have produced the 'Sheffield Risk and Treatment Tables' and these have been distributed to every GP in the UK. The tables are for primary prevention and use the more conservative 3% absolute risk level. The adoption of absolute rather than relative risk prioritizes older age groups. Younger patients with multiple risk factors may, by virtue of their age, not approach a 3% threshold.

The Sheffield tables have been criticized not only for their conservative absolute risk level but also because they omit data on family history and HDL cholesterol values. Patients from ethnic minorities or with genetic hyperlipidaemias are not well served and the extrapolations for diabetic or hypertensive women positively discourage cholesterol estimation.

Despite these reservations, the Standing Medical Advisory Committee (SMAC) in the UK has endorsed the use of the Sheffield tables for primary prevention in its guidelines on the use of statins (May 1997). People aged 35–69 without clinically apparent vascular disease who exceed a 3% risk level comprise 3.4% of the population (5.7% of men and 0.4% of women). A further 4.8% of the population (5.9% of men and 3.6% of women) already have overt atherosclerotic disease and form higher priority groups for intervention. In patients who have had a myocardial infarction, statin treatment is recommended when total cholesterol is as low as 4.8 mmol/l (LDL 3.23 mmol/l). In patients with angina, peripheral vascular disease or significant carotid disease and those who have had a bypass graft or

Figure 6.10
Guidelines for the management of hyperlipidaemia. Source: Pyörälä *et al.* (1994) Prevention of CHD in clinical practice: recommendations of the task force of the ESC, EAS and ESH. *European Heart Journal* **15** 1300–1331.

angioplasty, statin prescription is recommended from 5.5 mmol/l (LDL 3.7 mmol/l). These recommendations are extrapolated from CARE and 4S data, respectively.

Achieving targets

Achieving ideal targets can be very difficult. In the ASPIRE study (p. 217), amongst the minority of patients receiving lipid lowering medication in a secondary prevention context, over half failed to reach the BHA target level. In 4S, 28% failed to reach target LDL and data from the Simon Broome Trust (a register of FH patients in the UK) show average total cholesterol in treated patients to be 7.2 mmol/l.

Scoring systems in primary care

The appeal of scoring systems lies in devising an evidence-based method capable of stratifying risk which may act as a substitute for clinical judgment and may also have motivational influences for patients.

In 1986 the **Lifestyle Management Score** was produced, based on US data from the Pooling Project. Cholesterol levels from desktop analysers were computed by microprocessor with values for sex, family history, smoking, obesity and blood pressure. The method was designed for a nurse to give immediate feedback of the score to patients. Unfortunately the scores were unvalidated and non-predictive.

Also in 1986, **Shaper** devised scoring systems based on data applicable to middle-aged men from the British Regional Heart Study (p. 38). The contribution of each risk factor was established and numerically weighted to produce a score. The simplified formula for use in primary care is:

- $7 \times$ years of smoking;
- plus $6.5 \times$ mean BP;
- plus 270 if history of CHD;
- plus 150 if history of angina;
- plus 85 if either parent died from CHD;
- plus 150 if diabetic.

Scores in excess of 1000 identified the top 20% of the risk score distribution with a 53% prediction of those likely to have a CHD event in the next five years. A more sophisticated system including age, serum cholesterol and ECG parameters only improved the predictive capacity to 59%.

Criticisms of Shaper scoring include the fact that the data set was only drawn from men, that the role of cholesterol as a risk factor is under-estimated and that the system is prone to calculation errors.

The **Dundee Coronary Risk Disk** devised by Tunstall Pedoe in 1991 in Scotland is a circular double-disc slide rule which produces an age–sex-matched score for coronary risk based on smoking, systolic blood pressure and cholesterol. It does not include details of either personal or family history of CHD. The database was the UK Heart Disease Prevention Project (1973 – men only, aged 40–59 years) and it was validated against the Whitehall Study (male civil servants, aged 40–69 years) (Marmot *et al.*, 1991).

Those in the top 10% Dundee score distribution are six to seven times more likely to die of a fatal MI over the next five years than the bottom 10%. The Dundee Risk Disk can also calculate a rank from 1 to 100 (where 100 is lowest risk) which can indicate to a patient where they stand in a 'coronary queue'.

The Risk Disk is not immediately easy to use and, again, can be prone to calculation errors. Small changes in blood pressure or cholesterol measurement (both prone to measurement variation) can produce significant changes in score or rank, which can encourage or discourage a patient erroneously. Some assumptions are made regarding smoking cessation and the applicability to women is, again, questioned.

Scoring systems are still probably at an early stage and because they are difficult to use and complex, are rarely utilized in primary care.

Part Three
Intervention

Non-lipid risk factor modification

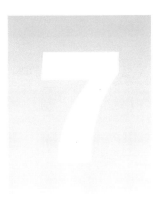

We have seen that the aetiology and assessment of CHD risk are multi-factorial. Modification of single risk factors to the exclusion of others is also inappropriate when it comes to treatment options.

Intervention strategies must include attention to lifestyle factors (smoking habit, exercise, obesity and alcohol) and the appropriate chronic management of hypertension and diabetes, as well as lipid modification with diet and drugs.

Changing people's habits

As health professionals begin to incorporate a preventive approach to their traditional curative/treatment roles, it becomes apparent that there is a requirement for new communication skills. In 1968 Davis demonstrated that patients only complied with 55% of their physician's advice. The receipt of adverse information such as a high serum cholesterol estimation can come as an initial shock to patients who feel well and high levels of fear can be paralysing. Holistic counselling can reduce fear to realistic levels to facilitate change. Primary health care teams need to be confident in their skills and this can only be fostered by training and support.

There are common threads to the facilitation of change:

1. **Elicit motivation.** This may be high in, for example, secondary prevention or families with bad histories of CHD but low in, for example, the recalcitrant smoker.
2. **Ascertain health beliefs.** It is important to know the patient's level of knowledge and interpretation of their position.
3. **Identify unhealthy influences.** Most habits are learned from an individual's experience in the community. Role models and peer group pressure are important – for example, teenage smoking. The keeping of diaries may help an individual to recognize associations with daily events leading to the possibility of behavioural modification.

4. **Persuasion**. It is often more effective to extol the positive benefits of change rather than the negative. For example, stopping smoking may lead to improved taste, smell, exertional tolerance and financial position as well as reduced disease risk.

5. **Planning and specific recommendation**. It is important that the individual retains 'control' and that agreed objectives (targets) are realistic and achievable. A gentle, structured change often increases motivation as success breeds positive reinforcement.

6. **Support and follow up**. Positive influences from health workers, friends, spouses, groups.

Cessation of smoking

Surveys have shown that large numbers of people would like to give up smoking. The most common reason for giving up is 'my doctor told me to' and yet only 22% of smokers recall their doctor advising them about their smoking habit.

In 1979, Russell showed that with firm advice to stop smoking, a leaflet and a warning of follow-up, 5.1% of smokers had stopped after one year. This rate has been confirmed on many occasions since. Even higher rates have been recorded in specialist smoking centres but the support and follow-up is much more intensive and the recruitment of very highly motivated patients may inflate their success. In the British Family Heart Study, a smoking cessation rate of 5% was recorded in men but it is disappointing that in the Oxcheck 4-year results there was no significant smoking reduction (p. 214).

It is hardly surprising that, with a failure rate of nearly 95%, primary health care teams feel despondent about smoking cessation and only 3% of GPs feel they are successful in helping patients to stop smoking. A 5% rate applied to all smokers, however, would result in about half a million fewer smokers per year and considerable health gain.

The collecting of health promotion data on smoking can provide a focus for discussion with the patient but there is better evidence for increased use of anti-smoking interventions when doctors and nurses have received quite minimal extra training.

NICOTINE REPLACEMENT THERAPY

The use of nicotine replacement using gum or adhesive patches may increase the cessation rates in self-referred, and therefore motivated, patients to approaching 15%. In the largest controlled trial in primary care, Russell in 1993 showed a cessation rate of 19.4% using patches compared with 11.8% using placebo in heavy smokers after three months. Unfortunately half had relapsed by the end of one year.

Nicotine gum (in 2 mg and 4 mg strengths) and three brands of nicotine patches are available over the counter but are not prescribable on the NHS in the UK. They offset the effects of nicotine withdrawal and are themselves slowly withdrawn over 8–12 weeks, most cravings subsiding by two months. A meta-analysis of 39 trials in 1994 showed an overall efficacy for the 2 mg gum of 6% whilst the efficacy of patches was 9%. Compliance was better with patches, which were deemed more convenient and socially acceptable. For high dependence smokers (high consumption, smoking within 30 minutes of waking), the 4 mg gum was effective at a rate of 16%. This probably represents the fact that gum can deliver a nicotine bolus to offset an acute craving, unlike the steady state delivery from a patch.

Cardiovascular diseases such as angina are often quoted as contra-indications to nicotine replacement but this is unwarranted as cigarette smoking itself is more detrimental. It is not advisable to use nicotine replacement in pregnancy.

Patches do cause itching and erythema and the process of withdrawal anyway often affects sleep and mood. Many young women are deterred from the average 4 kg weight gain that occurs on stopping smoking, though in terms of risk smoking is by far the more dangerous.

Nicotine nasal sprays and lozenges have been produced but some products are unlicensed and do not have substantiative trial data.

OTHER MEASURES

Acupuncture, hypnosis, relaxation training and meditation may all be useful adjuncts in some individuals to aid cessation of smoking. Effectiveness studies, however, unfortunately suffer from methodological problems.

Public health measures, including information and education, health warnings, bans on smoking in public places and reducing the tar content of cigarettes, are in existence. The sale of tobacco to children under 16 is banned in the UK, but this is hard to enforce. Most smokers start in adolescence and educational measures are of limited success in the face of the powerful role model provided by adult smokers.

Every 1% increase in taxation, however, produces a 0.5% drop in tobacco consumption. Tobacco advertising and promotion are powerful and millions are spent on campaigns, often linking smoking with sport and a glamourous lifestyle. A complete ban on advertising would potentially cut consumption by 6%.

THE RECALCITRANT SMOKER

If individuals have to smoke, they might be persuaded to smoke a lower tar cigarette and leave a longer butt. They might envisage non-smoking periods or locations – for example, not in front of children or in the car, etc. They may also be counselled to avoid situations they would naturally associate with smoking. Many smokers make several attempts before giving up, and continued encouragement and support will promote success.

Improving exercise

The benefits of exercise are multiple. Exercise aids weight reduction, increases HDL2 levels, increases insulin sensitivity, lowers blood pressure, improves coagulation factors and improves the psychological profile. People who exercise tend to smoke less than people who do not.

Aerobic exercise involves the repetitive movements of large muscle groups to induce cardio-respiratory training. Jogging, swimming, cycling and dancing will achieve this as well as fashionable exercise regimes. As an unsupervised exercise, particularly in older people, brisk walking will achieve adequate thresholds in up to two-thirds of patients. However, exercise needs to be a life-long pattern, enjoyable and convenient. If there is a social element, it is more likely to be repeated.

Exercise is monitored by heart rate. Ideally exercise should achieve 60–75% of a patient's maximum heart rate over 20–30 minutes if repeated 4–5 times per week, or over 45–60 minutes if repeated 2–3 times per week. Exercise sessions should be preceded by 5–10 minutes 'warm up' and followed by 5–10 minutes 'cool down'. A consensus conference of the National Institutes of Health in the United States (1996) recommended 30 minutes of moderate activity preferably every day. As a minimum, 20 minutes two or three times per week would suffice. Maximum heart rate is best estimated by exercise ECG testing but this is impractical and a rough approximation can be derived from subtracting the patient's age in years from 210.

Primary care doctors are often asked about the safety of exercise, particularly in those with pre-existing disease. Indeed, sanctioning of exercise by certification is often requested. An exercise ECG may be necessary for some patients to attest their fitness to exercise. Unlike isometric exercise, which can produce large rises in blood pressure, aerobic exercises are positively indicated for those with CHD provided a few simple rules are considered. For example, the dangers of exercise may be enhanced:

- in cold weather or after meals;
- with intercurrent illness, e.g. uncontrolled hypertension, viral infection;
- if symptoms emerge during exercise – feeling unwell, faint, chest pain, palpitations or excessive fatigue.

All regimes should follow a graded, progressive increase until cardio-respiratory fitness, based on frequency of exercise and pulse monitoring, is achieved. The patient should 'listen to the body' and report any adverse symptoms. Exercise must then be undertaken regularly, as unaccustomed or erratic exercise is hazardous.

Sensible drinking

In 1995 a consensus conference of UK physicians, psychiatrists and general practitioners reaffirmed previous medical evidence that men should drink no more than 21 units of alcohol a week and women no more than 14. In the light of research suggesting a reduction in CHD events for older men and post-menopausal women associated with moderate alcohol intake, the Department of Health in the UK has set 'benchmarks' for these groups of 3–4 units/day for men over 40 years old and 2–3 units/day for post-menopausal women. Unfortunately this advice may increase the problems associated with other co-morbid conditions associated with drinking more than 2 units per day and cannot be recommended as a serious strategy to prevent CHD.

As in smokers, simple advice from a primary health care team member can often be effective in reducing alcohol intake.

Control of hypertension

Primary care has rightly assumed the responsibility for the detection and management of most cases of hypertension within the population. The oft quoted 'Rule of Halves', however, stands as an indictment of the implementation of that responsibility, though there is considerable interpractice variation. The Rule of Halves suggests that only approximately half of the hypertensives in a given population are identified. Of those identified, only approximately half are treated and of those treated, only half achieve optimal blood pressure reduction.

The blame for this does not solely reside with primary care doctors. Whilst clinicians do vary in the levels of their knowledge, skills and beliefs in illness prevention, they are also influenced by cost–benefit considerations

Table 7.1
Treatment trials in elderly
hypertensive patients

Trial	Number in trial	% Reduction in CVA mortality	% Reduction in CHD mortality
EWPHE (1985) 60–97 years	840	32	38
Coope and Warrender (1986) 60–79 years	884	30	22
SHEP (1991) > 60 years	4736	36	27
STOP (1991) 70–84 years	1627	47	28
MRC (1992) 65–74 years	4396	25	19

and the possibility of inducing adverse effects through treatment in otherwise symptomless people. Patients, too, share differing health beliefs and may be poorly motivated to comply with treatment or follow-up.

Chapter 10 reproduces an example of locally produced 'end user' management guidelines commissioned to improve the quality of hypertension detection, diagnosis and management in primary care (see pp. 209–212). The guidelines are heavily based on the recommendations of the second working party of the British Hypertension Society. Emphasis is placed on:

- diagnosis in different age groups;
- the presence of coexisting risk factors or target organ damage as influences on intervention;
- non-pharmacological treatment;
- the 'tailoring' of pharmacological treatment to different patient profiles based on contraindications, side effects and the presence of coexisting disease.

In particular, the guidelines stress the recently published benefits in treating older people which are summarized in Table 7.1.

Control of diabetes

The prevalence of dyslipidaemia and atherosclerosis is increased in diabetics. In diabetic women, the usual protective effect of the female sex is lost. Apart from attention to glycaemic control, the management of hyperlipidaemia in diabetes requires attention to all risk factors and integrated approaches to cessation of smoking, dietary change, increasing exercise and the choice of appropriate anti-hypertensives when necessary. The excess risk of dyslipidaemia (often patterns of low HDL with raised triglyceride) may make lipid lowering with medication more appropriate.

Diet

Earlier chapters have suggested how changes in the current 'western' diet would confer benefits in CHD prevention at both population and individual levels. These changes can be summarized as:

- attainment of ideal body weight;
- reduction in intake of total fat, saturated fat and cholesterol;
- relative increase in intake of poly- and monounsaturated fats;
- increase in intake of unrefined carbohydrate;
- increase in intake of vitamin and mineral antioxidants;
- reduction in dietary sodium with an increase in potassium.

Attainment of ideal body weight

The body mass index (BMI) is calculated as a person's weight in kilograms divided by their height in metres, squared, and has become an accepted measure in the assessment of body weight (Figure 8.1). Optimal BMI is considered to be 20–25 kg/m^2 but 56% of UK males and 45% of UK females are currently overweight (> 25 kg/m^2) and 13% and 16%, respectively, are obese (> 30 kg/m^2), and these figures are rising.

If overweight, losing weight produces a drop in total cholesterol and triglyceride levels, and HDL cholesterol tends to rise. The effect is potent and there is no patient with hyperlipidaemia and obesity whose lipid levels would not benefit from weight loss.

In a survey of 20 000 people who lost weight (mean loss 15 kg), 72% achieved their weight loss alone, 20% employed commercial programmes and relatively few consulted health professionals. Whilst this underlines the fact that the responsibility for weight loss ultimately lies with the individual, the primary care team has much to offer in terms of advice, support and encouragement.

1. The **benefits** of weight loss can be illustrated in terms of improved appearance, effort tolerance, metabolic change (blood pressure, lipids and glucose) and increased life expectancy. In 1995 Williamson showed

Figure 8.1
Obesity: relationship between height and weight. Adapted from Garrow (1981).

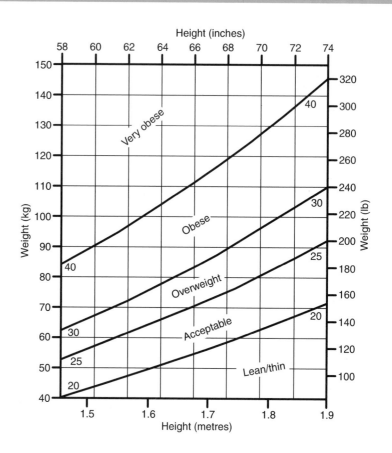

that in a group of 15 069 women with BMI > 27 and co-morbid conditions, **any** weight loss was associated with a 20% reduction in all-cause mortality.

2. **Targets** can be set encouraging a specific weight loss over a certain period. Targets should be flexible, with intermediate levels (perhaps 5–10% weight loss) when attainment of ideal body weight is a remote possibility. A loss of 0.5–1 kg per week is reasonable.

3. An **exercise regime** can be recommended. Whilst it takes a lot of exercise to lose only a little fat, lean body mass is maintained and there is improved morale and fitness.

4. **Follow-up** (weighing every 2–4 weeks) is essential to foster compliance and to motivate positively.

5. The **construction of a coherent plan** may involve no more than suggesting a change from inappropriate foods (fatty foods, sugar and alcohol) to more appropriate ones.

The **calorie-controlled diet** is the commonest weight-reducing strategy. This operates from the observation that excess weight is 75% fat and 25%

fat free tissue and has an energy value of 7000 kcal/kg. Therefore to lose 1 kg/week a person needs 1000 kcal negative balance per day. An average man requires 2500 kcal/day and an average woman 2100 kcal/day; therefore all obese people should lose weight on a diet of $<$ 1000 kcal/day and this is confirmed in controlled metabolic studies. The calorie-counting approach is limited by the need for meticulous measurement and recording and the ease of deception when faced with excess food which must be discarded.

'Crash diets' tend to achieve gratifying short-term loss but this is more at the expense of glycogen and water. Losses of greater than 1 kg/week (such as produced by Very Low Calorie Diets) tend to lose lean body mass as well as fat. Their use should be confined to periods of less than four weeks, their benefit being mainly motivational.

Many patients attend groups where the provision of structured plans, support and competition increases compliance. Simple behaviour modification techniques are used such as learning to eat more slowly or take smaller mouthfuls. Interestingly, men do well (in all male groups); women often achieve more weight loss with individual attention. For both men and women, 50–60% respond to the group approach, with average weight loss of 6–12 kg.

For some patients a lot of eating is automatic and bypasses critical analysis. For these people food diaries can provide information on patterns of eating, types of food, quantities and 'danger times' which may respond to modification.

Reduction in total fat

Whilst the consumption of fat in some countries with high rates of CHD has fallen, the amount of energy derived from fat in the UK still averages 38–42% of the total requirement, somewhat in excess of the ideal 30–35%.

Apart from making food more palatable, fat has physiological roles in the structure of every cell membrane, in the manufacture of steroids, prostaglandins and bile acids and as a major source of energy provision and storage. Fat is high in calories (9 kcal/g) compared with carbohydrate (4 kcal/g) and this is due to the extra oxygen atoms in carbohydrates and therefore less potential for oxidative respiration. Throughout nature, fat represents a high energy/low weight storage material, e.g. seed oils, keeping the seeds light and aiding dispersal.

During the second world war a deficiency of dietary energy led to a nutritional crisis in some countries. In Finland, Norway and Sweden the shortage of meat, eggs and butter correlated closely with a drop in CHD levels during the war years. In the UK the pre-war rise in CHD levelled off,

Figure 8.2

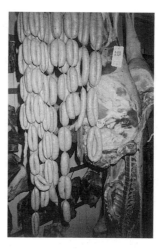

then resumed after the war; in the USA there was no change. High energy fat came to be viewed favourably and the impression that fat was good and carbohydrate bad lingered long after the war had ended. The ingenious variety whereby the food industry presents us fat in multiple disguises from sausages and paté, to pastry and cheeses, tempts us to choose by flavour rather than by required energy content (Figure 8.2). It is hardly surprising that, faced with nearly 2000 new products per year, little reduction in the fat content of the UK diet has occurred.

In 1973 the National Food Survey showed the percentage of energy derived from dietary fat to be 42% (50% saturated); 46% was derived from carbohydrate and 12% from protein. Whilst the consumption of saturated fats has stayed much the same, the consumption of polyunsaturated fats has risen.

FATTY ACID BIOCHEMISTRY

Fatty acids are formed from hydrocarbon chains with a **terminal methyl group** (CH_3) at one end and a **carboxyl group** (COOH) at the other. If there are no double bonds ($C=C$), the fatty acid is described as **saturated**.

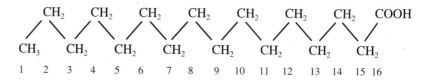

This is palmitic acid. There are 16 carbon atoms and no double bonds. It is noted C16 : 0.

If double bonds are present, the fatty acid is **unsaturated**. If one is present, it is **monounsaturated**; if more than one, **polyunsaturated**.

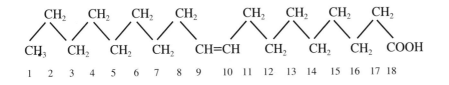

This is oleic acid (C18 : 1), a monounsaturated fatty acid.

The carbon of the terminal methyl group is called the **omega carbon** and the position of the double bond is counted from this (omega-9, or n-9).

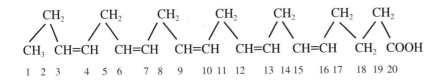

This is eicosapentaenoic acid (EPA) (C20 : 5), an omega-3 fatty acid. Omega-3 (n-3) describes the position of the double bond nearest the methyl group. Table 8.1 shows the major dietary fatty acids.

The hydrogen atoms bonded to the carbon atoms of the double bonds in unsaturated fatty acids normally lie on the same side of the double bond and *cis* isomers are formed (Figure 8.3). A kink is imparted to the hydrocarbon chain, which means that unsaturated fatty acids cannot pack closely together. The forces between them are less and their melting points correspondingly lower. This explains why vegetable oils rich in unsaturates are liquid at room temperature. Conversely, if the hydrogen atoms are on opposite sides of the double bond, the chains remain straight and *trans* isomers are formed (Figure 8.3). Saturated fatty acids are also straight and both they and *trans* fatty acids have higher melting points. This explains why saturated fat is solid at room temperature and so difficult to wash away after the Sunday roast.

Plants and cold-blooded animals can contain only those fatty acids that will remain liquid at the temperature of their habitat. Fish, for example, contain highly polyunsaturated fatty acids such as EPA and DHA (Table 8.1). Warm-blooded animals can tolerate saturated fats unless they live in cold habitats, in which case high levels of polyunsaturates are necessary to maintain fluidity – e.g. blubber of whales.

Table 8.1

Major dietary fatty acids

Structure	Fatty acid	Melting point (°C)
Saturated		
C 12 : 0	Lauric acid	44
C 14 : 0	Myristic acid	54
C 16 : 0	Palmitic acid	63
C 18 : 0	Stearic acid	70
Unsaturated		
Omega-9 (n-9)		
C 18 : 1 *cis*	Oleic acid	11
C 18 : 1 *trans*	Elaidic acid	45
Omega-6 (n-6)		
C 18 : 2	Linoleic acid	–5
Omega-3 (n-3)		
C 18 : 3	Linolenic acid	–11
C 20 : 5	Eicosapentaenoic acid (EPA)	–50
C 20 : 6	Docosahexaenoic acid (DHA)	–54

Figure 8.3

Cis and *trans* isomers of unsaturated fatty acids.

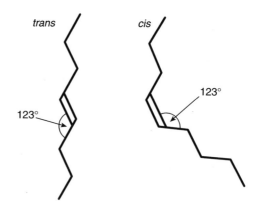

The percentage pattern of fatty acids in fats, oils and some meats in our diet is shown in Table 8.2. Whilst the proportions of fatty acids vary from food to food, no food is pure in fatty acid composition. Free use of a monounsaturate such as olive oil still adds saturates to the diet and so a reduction in total fat content in the diet is still required as well as a change in pattern.

Table 8.2
Percentage of fatty acids
in diet

Source	Saturated (C14–18)	Monounsaturated	Linoleic acid
Butter	69	28	3
Lamb	50	38	4
Beef	48	48	2
Palm oil	45	45	9
Pork	42	50	7
Hard margarine	37	33	12
Chicken	34	45	18
Soft margarine	21	22	52
Olive oil	14	73	11
Sunflower oil	12	33	58
Rapeseed oil	7	62	31

SATURATED FATTY ACIDS (SAFA)

Saturated fatty acids predominate in meat, butter, lard, hard margarine, suet and palm and coconut oils. They have the most significant effect on lipoproteins raising total cholesterol, LDL and triglyceride. Increased saturated fat intake was associated with increased CHD rates in the Seven Countries Study (p. 26).

Whilst C6–20 SAFA are found in the diet, C12–18 SAFA are the most prevalent: C16 (palmitic acid) is the commonest and C14 (myristic acid) the most hypercholesterolaemic. Short-chain (C10 or less) saturated fatty acids and C18 (stearic acid) seem to have no effect on lipoprotein levels, the latter being converted quickly into oleic acid in humans. This means that only three saturated fatty acids are atherogenic (C12, 14 and 16).

The proportion of dietary polyunsaturates to saturates is often expressed as the **P/S ratio** and used to describe the atherogenicity of a particular diet. As only three saturates are hypercholesterolaemic, this use of the ratio is technically inappropriate.

TRANS FATTY ACIDS (TFA)

Low levels of *trans* unsaturated fatty acids are present naturally in the diet, forming in ruminants and appearing in dairy products. Others are manufactured in the hardening of vegetable oils to produce margarine (hydrogenation). Their straight chains allow them to act like saturated fats and there is some evidence of a link with CHD from the Harvard Study of American Nurses. Metabolic studies show increased LDL and decreased

HDL and Holland has now banned *trans* fats from its margarines. Most major margarine manufacturers have also followed suit.

DIETARY CHOLESTEROL

Dietary cholesterol is mostly derived from dairy products, particularly eggs, but is also well known to originate from shellfish. It is incompletely absorbed from the gut (30–60%) and only exceeds 500 mg/day in diets already high in saturated fat. Halving this amount would have little impact on total cholesterol reduction (approximately 0.2 mmol/l) and attention to lowering dietary cholesterol is of major importance to few. Nevertheless, defiant stories of egg farmers who live to a hundred years old and of egg and prawn avoidance are rife. The confusion arises from a failure to understand that the diet to reduce the incidence of CHD is 'cholesterol lowering', not 'low cholesterol'.

MONOUNSATURATED FATTY ACIDS (MUFA)

Monounsaturated fatty acids are found in all animal products and vegetables. Particular sources include olive, rapeseed, avocado, most nuts, meat and peanut oil. The beneficial effects on lipoproteins were first described in 1957 but the observations were neglected for 30 years. When substituted for saturated fatty acids, total cholesterol, LDL and triglyceride are reduced and HDL either remains unchanged or slightly increased. The LDL produced appears lighter and less susceptible to oxidation.

The use of olive oil in Mediterranean countries over thousands of years provides strong epidemiological support for its use and safety.

POLYUNSATURATED FATTY ACIDS (PUFA)

Polyunsaturated fatty acids are found in vegetable oils, fish oils, most margarines, nuts and seeds – for example, sunflower, safflower, corn, sesame, soya and walnut oils. Coconut and palm oils tend to have more saturated fat than polyunsaturates. Linoleic acid is the commonest PUFA in the diet.

When substituting for saturates, polyunsaturated fatty acids lower total cholesterol, LDL and triglyceride more significantly than monounsaturates. Unfortunately they also produce a slight drop in HDL. Some polyunsaturates are essential to life as precursors of prostaglandins and prostacyclins.

Recently some concerns have emerged regarding the safety of polyunsaturates and these explain the switch of focus to monounsaturates as substitutes for saturates:

- No society has consumed high levels of omega-6 polyunsaturates for long enough to provide reassuring epidemiological evidence of safety.
- The slight reduction in HDL may be significant, particularly in women.
- LDL from people on a diet rich in linoleic acid seems to be more susceptible to oxidation.
- Animal experiments seem to suggest a decreased resistance to infection or neoplasia. This has not been verified in humans.
- The prevalence of gallstones is increased.
- Repeated reheating of polyunsaturated oil (e.g. a deep fat fryer) increases hydrogenation.

FISH OIL

Omega-3 polyunsaturates – eicosapentaenoic acid (EPA) and docosahex-aenoic acid (DPA) – are found particularly in oily fish such as sardines, pilchards, mackerel, herring, salmon, trout, halibut and tuna (not tinned). For example, 10 ml of cod-liver oil contains about 2 g of omega-3 fatty acids.

In 1927 attention was drawn to the apparently low rates of CHD in fish-eating communities such as Greenland Inuits (Eskimos). In recent years the accuracy of the mortality statistics have been questioned but in 1970 Danish scientists led an investigation into the dietary habits of Inuits. Compared with Danes or Inuits who had migrated to Denmark, native Inuits showed a slight reduction in serum cholesterol but a large 60% reduction in triglycerides. Dietary analysis using a double portion technique led to the discovery that the diet of native Inuits contained five times the level of omega-3 PUFAs than the diet of native Danes. The high levels of omega-3 polyunsaturates found in phytoplankton were being assimilated through the food chain by fish, whales and seals into the Inuit diet. In 1982 similar contrasts were found between Japanese fishermen and inland farmers.

Four prospective studies, including MRFIT, have all demonstrated the protective effect of fish consumption. Interestingly the findings in these studies also demonstrate the benefit of white fish in the diet. White fish is high in protein, vitamins and minerals and low in fat; it can act as a meat substitute and may have its own anti-thrombotic properties.

Much of the literature on diet and heart disease consists of reports of small feeding trials and there is a dearth of properly conducted randomized controlled trials. The only such trial of fish consumption is the Diet and Reinfarction Trial (DART – Burr, 1989). In this secondary prevention trial the study group assigned to eating oily fish twice weekly showed a surprising 29% reduction in all-cause mortality (33% reduction in CHD mortality).

If omega-3 fatty acids are ingested, the major effect is on triglyceride levels but at high dose total cholesterol may fall (10%) and HDL may rise. Fibrinogen is lowered, as is blood pressure, and there is reduced platelet aggregation. A reduction in atherosclerosis has been shown in four animal models.

EPA displaces arachidonic acid in platelets, reducing thromboxane synthesis and interfering with prostacyclin mechanisms, leading to reduced platelet aggregation. Prolonged bleeding times were confirmed in the Danish study and anecdotally Inuits were notorious for nosebleeds. Other anti-thrombotic effects are likely, particularly concerning vessel walls.

The therapeutic effect of fish oil supplements is considered later.

Dietary fibre

In 1975 Burkitt and Trowell presented their 'fibre hypothesis' linking low fibre intake in the diet to numerous western diseases, including CHD. Interest had again been stimulated by epidemiological considerations, in this case relating the high fibre diet of Africans (e.g. Ugandans eat 150 g/day) and their low rates of CHD. (The average fibre consumption in the UK is 20 g/day.)

Nowadays the term dietary fibre is misleading as it does not adequately describe some of the constituent indigestible non-starch carbohydrates, such as gums, that are included in the group. A better term is **non-starch polysaccharides**.

Non-starch polysaccharides can be divided into a water soluble fraction (pectin, gums, β-glucans) and an insoluble fraction (chiefly cellulose). The insoluble fraction (e.g. bread, pasta, breakfast cereals, brown rice and bran) has beneficial effects in preventing constipation and bowel disease but may only aid CHD prevention by having a substituting action for other more dangerous foods. In contrast, the soluble fraction found in pulses, oats, barley, nuts, seeds, fruit and vegetables excites interest because it has a cholesterol lowering effect.

Oatbran has been extensively studied and in 1987 a book extolling its virtues, *The Eight Week Cholesterol Cure*, sold 2 million copies. Cereal manufacturers produced heart-shaped bowls and much advertising centred on the observation that eating 60–100 g/day would reduce cholesterol by 5%. Unfortunately an average cereal bowl contains only 30–40 g and therefore the amounts used were large and not practical. Pectin and guar gum also lower cholesterol (guar gum by 15%) but again the amounts used are too large and unpalatable.

Oats contain β glucan, which forms a viscous non-starch polysaccharide in the gut that delays bile acid reabsorption. This leads to increased bile acid output and the excess bile acids are sequestered by colonic bacteria. Insulin secretion is reduced if oatbran is given with a meal. A third mechanism may just involve substitution: if you eat lots of oats you may have no room left for the bacon and eggs. It is ironic that the countries with the highest oat consumption in the world are Scotland and Finland, both renowned for their high rates of CHD.

The Diet and Reinfarction Trial also investigated the effect of fibre, but using cereal fibre that was largely wheat based. No benefit was found and a randomized controlled trial of soluble fibre is needed.

There is little evidence that simple refined carbohydrates such as sucrose promote CHD; indeed Cuba, with the highest per capita sucrose consumption in the world, has low rates of CHD. Sucrose may, however, increase obesity and raise triglycerides, and of course it promotes tooth decay.

Antioxidants

Respiration depends on oxygen to release energy to drive all bodily functions. The notion that oxygen may be harmful to us is not immediately apparent. The reduction of oxygen to form water involves the addition of four electrons and the potential formation of the potent oxidizing agent OH· – the free hydroxyl radical. Oxygen radicals can react with lipids (producing oxidized LDL or structural phospholipid damage), with protein (producing cross-linking and degradation) and with DNA (producing errors and deletions). Thus free radicals may be implicated in the processes of cardiovascular disease, cancer and ageing.

Antioxidants exist to trap free radicals and render them inert and many substances have been described. Enzymes with trace elements (selenium, copper, manganese and zinc) and vitamin E (α-tocopherol), vitamin C (ascorbic acid) and β-carotene (a precursor of vitamin A) are all examples. In animal models, 15 out of 18 studies show that antioxidants slow the progression of atherosclerosis. There is intense interest in the properties of these 'neutraceuticals' but the evidence of benefit is inconsistent.

Vitamin E is commonly found in foods high in polyunsaturates, and it is the substance in vegetable oil that prevents it oxidizing (going rancid). It is the most abundant antioxidant in plasma and this may reflect its importance. Three studies have found no benefit from **vitamin E** ingestion but in 1993 published surveys of American doctors and nurses showed significant reductions in CHD in users of vitamin E supplement (100 mg). As the supplement users may be generally healthier individuals, these studies may be confounded. In Scotland, low vitamin E levels were found in the plasma of newly diagnosed angina patients.

Experimental data on **vitamin C** suggests small falls in cholesterol, LDL oxidation, fibrinogen and blood pressure.

Low levels of β-**carotene** are found in patients with myocardial infarction and in smokers. A small subset of the Physicians Health Study (designed to prevent cancer with β-carotene) suggested a reduction of CHD events of 44%. The need for caution is highlighted by the finding that β-carotene supplementation in Finnish smokers increased the risk of lung cancer (CARET, 1996).

There has been considerable interest in dietary **flavonoids** probably due to the fact that apart from being found in fruits, vegetables and tea, red wine is a good source. *In vitro* studies confirm that flavonoids are powerful inhibitors of the oxidation of LDL. A 26-year follow-up study from Finland published in 1996 suggests increased levels of CHD where dietary flavonoids are low, the prime sources in Finland being apples and onions. Generally, however, the evidence that flavonoids protect against CHD is inconsistent.

With all the antioxidants, where epidemiological evidence suggests a link there is a need for clinical trials. The Cambridge Heart Antioxidant Study (CHAOS) (Stephens *et al.*, 1996) was a secondary prevention study of 2002 patients taking high dose vitamin E (400–800 mg) but with only a short follow-up period of 17 months. Non-fatal MI was reduced by 77% but there was no reduction in overall cardiovascular mortality and the trial raised more questions than it answered. An earlier trial using 50 mg vitamin E in lung cancer prevention failed to show any reduction in CHD.

Until further clinical trials have been published, it seems reasonable to increase consumption of fruit and vegetables which abound in antioxidants and a recent campaign extols the virtues of five portions a day (Table 8.3).

Sodium and potassium

There is abundant evidence that high dietary sodium and low dietary potassium are causally related to raised blood pressure. Reducing sodium and increasing potassium by 40 mmol/day would result in a drop of 2–6 mm Hg. Over the population a 2 mm drop in BP would result in a 5% reduction in CHD and 11% reduction in CVA. Avoiding visible salt and processed foods (food processing increases sodium content and reduces potassium) together with one or two extra servings of fruit or vegetables is sufficient.

In Finland, where intensive cardiovascular programmes have raised life expectancy by seven years over the last two decades, alteration in dietary

Type	Example	Portion
Fruit		
Very large	Melon, pineapple	1 large slice
Large	Apple, banana	1 whole
Medium	Plum, kiwi	2 whole
Berries	Raspberries, grapes	1 cupful
Stewed/canned	Stewed apple/tinned peaches	3 serving spoonfuls
Dried	Dried apricots	$\frac{1}{2}$ serving spoonful
Fruit juice	Orange juice	full wine glass
Vegetables		
Green	Broccoli, spinach	2 serving spoonfuls
Root	Carrots, parsnip	2 serving spoonfuls
Small	Peas, sweetcorn	3 serving spoonfuls
Salad	Lettuce, tomato	1 bowlful
Pulses	Beans	2 serving spoonfuls

Table 8.3
'Five portions a day': what is a portion?

electrolytes is identified as probably the biggest responsive factor. A modified table salt, 'Pansuola', has been introduced with the composition: 57% NaCl, 28% KCl, 12% $MgSO_4$, 2% L-lysine, KI and anticaking agent. Using Pansuola, sodium intake is reduced by 30–50% with improvement in the sodium:potassium ratio. The taste and properties of Pansuola are acceptable and food manufacturers in the UK are beginning to incorporate it into some products.

Other dietary factors

COFFEE

Strong relationships between heavy coffee drinking (more than 5 cups/day) and CHD have been described in Scandinavian countries and parts of North America. The interpretation of these findings is difficult, as heavy coffee drinkers are often heavy smokers, but La Croix showed that amongst American doctors (largely non-smokers) there was a 2–3-fold increased risk of CHD in heavy consumers. In Norway differences of up to 0.79 mmol/l in men and 0.72 mmol/l in women were found between the highest and lowest consumers. In Italy, where coffee is filtered rather than boiled, the differences were more modest, of the order of 0.25 mmol/l.

It is proposed that the preparation of coffee by boiling releases substances (the diterpenes cafestol and kahweol have been identified) that probably stimulate LDL synthesis. Experiments where coffee oil has been added surreptitiously to the diet have increased LDL by 29%. Filtering coffee, using decaffeinated coffee or granules, has much less adverse effect.

GARLIC

The medicinal properties of garlic (*Allium sativum*) have been recognized since Egyptian times and garlic is often to be found in Mediterranean cuisine. Preparations of garlic are the biggest selling over-the-counter drugs in Germany and it has been promoted as 'the world's most ancient, versatile and enjoyable medicine' The active ingredients are organo sulphur compounds (hence the smell) and crushing a clove releases enzymes which form allicin from odourless alliin. Other metabolites may be important and both they and allicin are refined with considerable variation into several commercial products.

Claims are made that garlic will reduce cholesterol, LDL, triglycerides, blood pressure, fibrinogen and platelet aggregation and increase HDL and vessel flow. Many studies are poorly conducted and a recent meta-analysis that showed an overall reduction of 0.5 mmol/l in serum cholesterol may have suffered from publication bias. In 1989 Kleijnen suggested that whilst 7–28 cloves/day may help, the data for commercial preparations was less convincing. In 1990 a double-blind controlled trial was conducted in Germany which showed reductions of 11.7% and 17% in total cholesterol and triglycerides, respectively. It is significant that 21% of the participants reported the observation of odour. In contrast, a well conducted trial from British general practice (Neil, 1996) found no significant differences in lipid concentrations after six months between treatment and control groups.

The mechanisms whereby garlic exerts its cardiovascular benefit are unknown but it is interesting to note that extracts of garlic other than allicin have been found to inhibit HMG CoA reductase.

SITOSTEROL

In Finland, Miettinen *et al.* converted the plant sterol, sitosterol, into sitosterol ester, a compound that has a significant cholesterol-lowering effect. As a 10% suspension in margarine ('Benecol'), LDL was lowered by 13%.

Patterns of eating

The Oxford Vegetarian Study is a prospective study of 6000 subjects who do not eat meat and 5000 meat-eating controls. The meat eaters have a blood cholesterol near the UK average (5.9 mmol/l) with lower levels for fish eaters (5.6 mmol/l) and vegetarians (5.3 mmol/l), and lowest of all for vegans (5.0 mmol/l). Several studies from Britain and California show that CHD mortality is reduced in vegetarians by about 30%.

There is some evidence too that the way in which we eat may influence cholesterol levels. 'Nibbling' or 'grazing' is associated with a reduction of 8.5% when compared with 'gorging'.

Diet strategies

> I want to buy some real farmhouse butter, some real farmhouse eggs and some clotted cream – and I am not going to listen to those dietary faddists who say don't eat it.
>
> Margaret Thatcher. *The Independent*, 1987

Many august bodies have produced diet strategies. In the UK the Committee on Medical Aspects of Food Policy (COMA, Table 8.4) and the UK National Advisory Committee on Nutrition Education (NACNE), and in the United States the National Cholesterol Education Programme (NCEP) and the Adult Treatment Panel (ATP) have all issued reports. The diet recommendations of the European Atherosclerosis Society (EAS) are shown in Table 8.5.

	SAFA	PUFA	MUFA	TFA
Recommended	≤ 10	6	15	≤ 2
UK average	16	6	15	2

Table 8.4
COMA (Committee on Medical Aspects of Food Policy) recommended and average percentage contribution of fatty acids to diet in UK, 1994

In the UK much progress is needed to achieve the dietary targets of the Health of the Nation initiative by the year 2005.

Issuing dietary strategies in percentage terms leads to a problem in interpretation for primary care team members, very few of whom are well versed in aspects of nutrition. Not many health professionals can identify what percentage of their day's energy has been derived from saturated fat.

Principle	Amount	Food sources
Decreased total fat Decreased saturated fat	< 30% energy 7% to 10% of energy	Avoid butter, hard margarine, whole milk, cream, ice cream, high fat cheese, fatty meats and poulty, sausages, pastries, coffee whitener, products containing hydrogenated oils, palm oil and coconut oil
Increased use of high protein food (low in saturated fat)		Fish, chicken and turkey, veal, game, spring lamb
Increased complex carbohydrate; increased fruit and vegetable fibre; increased legumes	About 35 g/day of fibre, one-half derived from fruit and vegetables	All fruit, including dried fruit, all fresh and frozen vegetables; lentils, dried beans, chick peas; unrefined cereal foods, including oats
Decreased dietary cholesterol	< 300 mg/day	Allowance up to 2 egg yolks per week and liver up to twice monthly; other offal avoided
Moderately increased use of mono- and polyunsaturated oils and products	Mono: 10% to 15% of energy Poly: 7% to 10% of energy	Olive oil, sunflower oil, corn oil and products based on these

Table 8.5
Dietary recommendations of the European Atherosclerosis Society (EAS, 1992, *Nutrition, Metabolism and Cardiovascular Diseases*, **2**, 113–156)

With fewer than 1500 state-registered dieticians in the UK NHS, most of whom are hospital based, there is a need to expand the profession. More education is necessary, not only for health professionals but also in the workplace, schools and ethnic communities.

The effect of diet on serum lipids

The effect of dietary factors on serum lipids is summarized in Table 8.6.

Compliance with a cholesterol-lowering diet is commonly associated with a reduction in serum cholesterol of 10–15%. Reductions up to 20% can be obtained if the diet is more rigid and possibly even greater if weight loss is involved. Truswell's (1994) review of 17 dietary intervention studies showed that the odds ratio of intervention versus control groups was 0.94 for total deaths and 0.87 for coronary events. The effects of the dietary change maximize after several months and this means that diet alone can often be

Dietary component	Total cholesterol	LDL	HDL	TG
Saturated fats	↑↑	↑↑	↑	↑↑
Omega-3 polyunsaturates	↓	↓	↑→	↓↓
Omega-6 polyunsaturates	↓↓	↓↓	↓	
Monounsaturates	↓	↓	↑→	↓
Dietary cholesterol	↑	↑	↑	
Soluble fibre	↓	↓		
Alcohol			↑	↑↑
Excess calories	↑↑	↑↑	↓	↑↑

Table 8.6
Effect of dietary factors on serum lipids

successful in controlling hyperlipidaemia. Dietary change, even with full compliance, is less effective for some, – for example, those with genetic hyperlipidaemias – but good diet enhances the effect of drugs if they are required (Table 8.7). The reader will recall the significance of a 10% drop in serum cholesterol from the Cholesterol Papers (Law *et al.*) (p. 42).

Dietary studies are often criticized because community studies, with free-living subjects, are potentially unreliable and experimental 'metabolic ward' studies are often too small. In 1991 Ramsey *et al.* re-opened the debate on the efficacy of cholesterol lowering by diet. They divided 16 published trials of dietary intervention into NCEP Step 1 and more rigorous diet groups. The NCEP had recommended a two-step dietary approach: Step 1 for the general public and for most people under treatment, Step 2 for more severe cases of hypercholesterolaemia (Table 8.8).

In Ramsey's analysis the Step 1 study group showed an average fall of only 2% in serum cholesterol whereas the more rigorous diet group showed up to 15.5% reduction. The analysis achieved notorious publicity ('Hole in the Heart of the Cholesterol Cult' – *The Times*) but has been criticized on several counts:

Diet	Total cholesterol (mmol/l)	
	Diet alone	Diet + simvastatin
High fat	9.6	7.6
Low fat	7.8	6.3

Table 8.7
Effects of dietary change with and without medication

Table 8.8
NCEP (National Cholesterol
Education Program, USA)
two-step dietary approach

Dietary factor	Step 1	Step 2
Total fat	< 30%	< 30%
SAFA	< 10%	< 7%
PUFA	10–15%	10–15%
MUFA	< 10%	< 10%
P/S ratio	1.0	1.4
Cholesterol	300 mg/day	200 mg/day

- The diets in the more rigorous group are not significantly different from those in the Step 1 group. For example, in the Oslo Study (p. 57) included in the second group, total fat was 28%, P/S ratio 1.01 and cholesterol 289 mg/day. The Oslo trial was well conducted on free-living men over a period of five years and showed serum cholesterol reduction of 13% and a reduction of MI and sudden death by 47%.
- The population effect in control groups (eg MRFIT; see p. 37) was discounted.
- Compliance with some of the diets of the Step 1 group was suboptimal.
- The common experience of most clinicians is that many patients show significant reductions in serum cholesterol with diet alone.

The relative contributions of dietary factors to reducing serum cholesterol can be summarized as:

- Major effects:
  - weight loss;
  - reducing the amount and saturation of fat;
  - avoiding boiled coffee.
- Lesser effects;
  - reducing dietary cholesterol;
  - increasing soluble fibre;
  - garlic;
  - meal patterns.

Practical advice

Rather than include diet sheets which by their long lists of negatives can be intimidating, members of the primary care team can learn a series of simple dietary messages to impart to patients. (The advice, though, is practical for all.) Here are ten simple dietary measures to avoid CHD:

- Optimize body weight.
- Eat lean meat and discard excess fat.
- Change milk to skimmed/semi-skimmed.
- Use soft margarines, thinly spread.
- Select low fat cheeses.
- Eat fish twice a week (especially oily fish).
- Increase fruit and vegetables (five portions/day).
- Use liquid vegetable oils for cooking (especially MUFA).
- Filter coffee.
- Maintain sensible alcohol limits.

Patients should be encouraged to look at their sources of fat and scrutinize food labels. Unfortunately food labelling is often misleading, fat content being described as grams of fat/100g. A pork pie, for example, may contain 25% fat by weight but 75% of the energy of the pie may be supplied from fat once the water content is removed.

Alternative cooking methods – grilling, boiling, baking, steaming, poaching, microwaving, casseroling, using the barbecue or the stir fry – can reduce the fat content of our diet.

People in the UK eat on average three meals per week out of the home and this can upset the best of plans. Even foreign menus have become

---

	Table 8.9
1. Use straight-cut, thick chips. Thin or crinkle-cut chips increase the surface area and therefore the absorption of fat.	Five tips for low fat chips
2. Use vegetable oil high in PUFA or MUFA. With PUFA, remember to change the oil after every use.	
3. Seal the chips in preheated fat to limit the amount of fat absorbed.	
4. Do not use chips straight from the freezer. This cools the oil, preventing sealing and increasing fat absorption.	
5. When cooked, blot the chips dry on kitchen paper towel to remove excess fat.	
Chips prepared in this way contain less than 5% fat – far from ideal but an illustration of compromise by alteration of preparation method.	

anglicized and it may be better to have fish and chips fried in vegetable oil (Table 8.9) rather than doner kebabs or Indian take-aways.

A patient's diet should also be discussed in the context of the rest of the family, shopping facilities and financial constraints.

No diet that is dull, uninteresting or unpalatable will secure compliance and cholesterol-lowering diets have this reputation. The variety of flavour and appearance in the diet of many Mediterranean countries, however, proclaims the reverse and with proper advice and imagination we can all receive the cardiovascular benefit of a healthier diet.

Lipid-lowering drugs

In recent years major new therapeutic agents have been added to available lipid-lowering drugs such that goals of therapy can be achieved in the majority of patients. In most cases this will be possible with mono-therapy; others, particularly the more severe monogenic disorders, will require combination therapy.

In this section the available classes of lipid-lowering drugs will be discussed in detail. Where significant differences are apparent between individual drugs of a particular class, these will be highlighted. It is convenient to consider the various drug classes as those that primarily lower cholesterol concentrations, those that primarily lower triglyceride concentrations and those that lower both cholesterol and triglycerides.

Cholesterol-lowering drugs

BILE ACID SEQUESTRANTS

These drugs have been available for many years (cholestyramine was introduced in 1967) and considerable clinical experience has accumulated from extensive well-conducted clinical trials, including end-point studies. They have a major advantage in that they are not absorbed and therefore do not have the potential to produce toxic side-effects. Major disadvantages are that some patients find them tiresome and inconvenient to take and the frequency of gastrointestinal side-effects. The available compounds are cholestyramine and colestipol. As there are no clinically important differences between the two agents, they will be considered together.

Mechanism of action
Cholestyramine is a copolymer of styrene and divinyl benzene; colestipol is a copolymer of diethylpentamine and epichlorohydrin. Unabsorbed after oral administration, they bind bile acids in the intestinal lumen – interrupting the entero-hepatic circulation. As a result, the faecal loss of bile

acids and cholesterol is increased, which leads to compensatory changes in hepatic metabolism. The conversion of cholesterol to bile acids is stimulated through activation of the enzyme 7αhydroxylase, which catalyses the rate-determining step in bile acid synthesis. As hepatic cholesterol content is reduced through this process there is up-regulation LDL receptor activity, enhanced hepatic extraction of LDL from the circulation and decreased plasma LDL cholesterol concentrations. Part of the ability of resins to up-regulate LDL receptor activity is offset, because hepatic cholesterol synthesis is also stimulated through increased activity of HMG CoA reductase, which catalyses the rate-determining step in cholesterol metabolism.

Pharmacology and clinical efficacy

The major effect is to reduce LDL cholesterol. The effect is maximal at about two weeks. After discontinuation, LDL levels return to baseline after three to four weeks. A small increase in HDL cholesterol is usually observed, though the mechanism of this effect is not understood. During the first few weeks of therapy there is often a transient increase in VLDL triglyceride (5–20%) which generally reverts to baseline levels after two to three months. This effect is more pronounced in individuals with pre-existing hypertriglyceridaemia.

At moderate doses (cholestyramine 16 g/day; colestipol 20 g/day) LDL cholesterol reductions of 15–30% can be expected in hypercholesterolaemic individuals already on dietary measures. Reported increases in triglyceride concentrations range between 5 and 15%. Several studies have been performed in heterozygous FH and similar results on LDL cholesterol have been observed. With good compliance the effects on LDL cholesterol are maintained in the long term. In FH patients regression of tendon xanthomata has been observed.

Cholestyramine was used in an important early primary prevention trial – the Lipid Research Clinics Coronary Primary Prevention Trial (LRC, CPPT). In this randomized, double-blind study involving 3806 hyper-cholesterolaemic (> 6.8 mmol/l) men, LDL reduction with cholestyramine over an average 7.4 years of follow-up was associated with a significant reduction in definite CHD death and/or non-fatal myocardial infarction. Subsequently both cholestyramine and colestipol have been used, either alone or in combination with other lipid-lowering agents in angiographic trials, with beneficial effects (p. 74).

Adverse effects

Cholestyramine and colestipol are administered as powders. The powder is either scooped from a tin with a measured spoon or provided in sachets (cholestyramine 4 g; colestipol 5 g). The powders are mixed well with water or juice and are taken before a meal. The powder can also be sprinkled on food. These procedures are clearly a nuisance in comparison with simple tablet taking and patients often complain about the resins' gritty texture.

The adverse effects are more annoying than serious but do make a considerable impact on compliance. The main complaints are of constipation, a bloated feeling, flatulence, heartburn and nausea in up to a quarter of patients.

The resins can interfere with the absorption of other drugs. It is important that resins are taken either one hour before or four hours after other medications. In very high doses, malabsorption of fat may occur with decreased absorption of fat-soluble vitamins, and hypoprothrombinaemia has been described. Vitamin supplements may be required with prolonged high dosage. The gastrointestinal side-effects of resins tend to ameliorate with prolonged use. Patient disenchantment at the initiation of treatment can be partly overcome by low dosage (half a sachet daily) with a gradual increase over 4–6 weeks. Some patients mix the whole of their daily dose the day before and refrigerate it overnight, as they find the texture becomes more acceptable.

Various alternative preparations have been made available in some countries to try to improve compliance, e.g. tablet forms and chewy fruit-flavoured bars. However, in our experience these preparations do not offer any striking advantages.

Indications

The resins are indicated for the treatment of isolated primary hypercholesterolaemia. In mixed lipaemia they can be combined with a fibrate or nicotinic acid. In severe hypercholesterolaemia they can be combined with an HMG CoA reductase inhibitor. It is our current practice to use low dose therapy (2 sachets/day) for mild to moderate hypercholesterolaemia in individuals who have concerns about systemically active drugs. The resins are particularly useful in children and in women of child-bearing potential.

PROBUCOL

This lipophilic bis-phenol compound with strong antioxidant properties was demonstrated to have a cholesterol-lowering effect in the late 1960s. It has never achieved more than second or third line status as a lipid-lowering drug. It is only modestly effective in reducing cholesterol. Furthermore, some of the reduction in total cholesterol is due to a reduction in HDL cholesterol.

Mechanism of action

The mode of action is not fully understood, but it appears that probucol increases the fractional catabolic rate of LDL but through non-LDL receptor pathways. This probably explains why the drug produces a modest cholesterol reduction in patients with homozygous familial hypercholesterolaemia who do not possess normal LDL receptors. Through its antioxidant properties probucol can reduce the oxidative modification of LDL and in animals it has been shown to have an anti-atherosclerotic effect.

Pharmacology and clinical efficacy

Probucol is relatively poorly absorbed with subsequent low bio-availability. It is highly lipophilic with a long elimination half-life, such that detectable concentrations may persist in patients for up to six months after administration is stopped.

LDL cholesterol is reduced by about 15% with probucol treatment and with similar or greater reductions in HDL, probably through inhibition of apoprotein A-I synthesis. The drug has no effect on triglycerides.

Probucol has not been used in a primary or secondary prevention study of CHD. It was used in an angiographic study of atherosclerosis progression/regression in the femoral arteries but no effect was observed, which is disappointing given its effect in experimental models of atherosclerosis. When combined with an HMG CoA reductase inhibitor, more marked effects were observed in restoring coronary artery endothelial function *in vivo* compared with the HMG CoA reductase inhibitor alone.

Adverse effects

Probucol is generally well tolerated but can produce diarrhoea in about 10% of patients, together with other gastrointestinal effects, nausea, flatulence and abdominal pain. These effects become less marked with time. Prolongation of the QT interval on the ECG can occur and therefore probucol is best avoided in patients at risk of ventricular arrhythmias. Because of the very long elimination time due to persistence of the drug in adipose tissue, effective contraception should not be withdrawn for at least six months after stopping the drug.

Indications

Probucol had a licence for the treatment of hypercholesterolaemia and the recommended dosage is 500 mg bd. It did not play a significant part in our therapeutic choices. Probucol has recently been withdrawn in the UK and other countries and is no longer available for clinical use.

Triglyceride-lowering drugs

OMEGA-3 FISH OILS

Fish oils rich in the omega-3 fatty acids, eicosapentaenoic acid (EPA) and docosahexaenoic acid (DHA), have a limited but useful place in the therapy of lipid disorders. Interest in fish oils stemmed from epidemiological studies which contrasted the plasma lipid levels of Greenland Inuits and Danes. Despite the high fat diet of the Inuits, their plasma triglyceride levels were lower. If non-Inuits were fed the Inuit diet, with a large percentage of calories derived from oily fish, reductions in plasma triglycerides were observed.

Mechanism of action

Fish oils reduce plasma triglyceride by reducing hepatic VLDL triglyceride synthesis. At very high doses VLDL apoprotein B secretion is also reduced, with reductions of plasma cholesterol. At lower doses, although triglyceride levels are reduced, LDL cholesterol may increase – possibly through enhanced conversion of VLDL to LDL. HDL cholesterol remains largely unchanged.

Pharmacology and clinical efficacy

In some countries, including the UK, a fish oil preparation is licensed for use in the treatment of severe hypertriglyceridaemia. Maxepa (gelatin capsules or liquid) contain 18% by weight of EPA and 12% by weight of DHA.

The recommended dosage is 10 capsules a day in divided doses or 5 ml twice daily of the liquid form. At these doses triglyceride concentrations will be reduced by 50–60% in severely hypertriglyceridaemic patients. LDL cholesterol concentrations, which are low in these patients, tend to rise.

Fish oil administration has not been subjected to a long-term, randomized, controlled clinical trial with hard CHD end-points. However, dietary measures to increase the consumption of fatty fish were associated with a significant reduction in CHD death in post-myocardial infarction patients.

Adverse effects

Although a 'natural' product, it cannot be assumed that the long-term consumption of fish oils at pharmacological doses will be harmless. Nevertheless the intake of omega-3 fatty acids by some population groups throughout the world probably approaches the equivalent of Maxepa 10 g/day with no apparent untoward effects. The most common side effects are nausea and eructation.

Polyunsaturated fatty acids such as the omega-3 acids have numerous double bonds (EPA has five and DHA has six) which theoretically are at risk of attack by free radicals with formation of lipid peroxides, which are toxic. For this reason it is important to increase the consumption of antioxidants. In Maxepa capsules d-α-tocopheryl acetate is added as an antioxidant.

Indications

Maxepa is useful for the treatment of severe hypertriglyceridaemia and the authors often use it in combination with a fibrate drug. In patients with mixed hyperlipidaemia with more modest elevations of triglyceride concentration, some patients respond well to a combination of fish oil with an HMG CoA reductase inhibitor. Fish oil should not be used alone in these patients because of the increase in LDL cholesterol.

We have used Maxepa successfully in women with familial hypertriglyceridaemia at risk of pancreatitis during pregnancy.

More research is needed on the optimal dosing for fish oil supplementation together with end-point trials. The potential of omega-3 fatty acids to influence other important processes in atherogenesis and thrombosis (e.g. platelet function and vascular tone) is exciting.

Drugs that lower cholesterol and triglyceride

NICOTINIC ACID (NIACIN)

Altschul and colleagues in the 1950s first demonstrated that nicotinic acid could reduce plasma lipids. This effect is independent of its action as a vitamin and is only observed at high dose. Importantly its amide derivative, nicotinamide (vitamin B_3) is ineffective.

There is no doubt that in terms of its broad spectrum of effect in modulating plasma lipid and lipoprotein concentrations, nicotinic acid could be considered to be the ideal drug. Sadly its wider use is markedly restricted because of poor patient acceptability and metabolic side effects.

Mechanism of action

Kinetic studies have shown that the major effect is to reduce hepatic output of VLDL with consequent reductions in IDL and LDL. The increase in HDL (often pronounced) seen with nicotinic acid is most marked in hypertriglyceridaemic individuals and is due to decreased clearance of the lipoprotein. It is known that HDL clearance is enhanced in hyper-triglyceridaemia and the reduction in plasma triglycerides by nicotinic acid appears to correct this.

Whilst the reduction in VLDL output is clear the cellular mechanisms underlying this effect remain to be explained. It is not only VLDL triglyceride that is reduced, its protein components – apoprotein B, C and E – are all reduced.

Nicotinic acid inhibits hormone-sensitive lipase in adipose tissue with consequent reduction of free fatty acid flux to the liver. As this is a major determinant of VLDL output it is attractive to hypothesize that this is the major explanation for nicotinic acid's effect. However, this effect is relatively short term. Two to three hours after dosing, free fatty acid concentrations are back to baseline and continue to rise with a significant overshoot, whilst triglyceride concentrations may remain reduced for 12–24 hours.

Nicotinic acid is unique amongst current lipid-modifying drugs, in that it reduces lipoprotein(a), but the mechanism of this effect is unknown.

Pharmacology and clinical efficacy

For effective reduction of plasma cholesterol and triglyceride, doses of nicotinic acid in the region of 2–8 g/day are required. At this dosage, reductions of total cholesterol of up to 30% are to be expected, and LDL cholesterol concentrations fall by a similar amount. Reductions in plasma triglyceride vary depending on baseline levels. If triglyceride concentrations are in the normal range then small decreases ($\simeq 20\%$) are usual, but in hypertriglyceridaemic patients reductions of up to 60% are not uncommon. It is of interest that increases in HDL cholesterol may be observed with lower doses (1 g/day). Nicotinic acid is particularly effective in increasing HDL cholesterol concentrations in hypertriglyceridaemic patients; increases of up to 30% are not uncommon and occasionally increases of 50% are observed.

Nicotinic acid is highly effective in patients with dysbetalipoproteinaemia and reductions in remnant particles of 50–60% are to be expected.

In patients with elevated LDL and/or VLDL, nicotinic acid at a dose of 4 g/day reduces lipoprotein(a) concentrations; the most marked effect (a reduction of 38%) has been observed in hypertriglyceridaemic patients.

Nicotinic has been used alone or in combination as the therapeutic agent in two secondary prevention trials and several angiographic progression/regression trials. In the Coronary Drug Project, nicotinic acid (3 g/day) was one of the five treatment arms, with 1119 men (aged 30–64 years) randomized to receive the drug. A placebo group consisted of 2789 men. In the nicotinic acid treated group, sustained reductions in total cholesterol of 10% and in triglycerides of 26% were achieved. After five years a significant reduction was observed in definite non-fatal myocardial infarction, but there was no difference in cardiovascular death or overall mortality. When the vital status of the study participants was ascertained nine years after the completion of the study, mortality in the group treated with nicotinic acid was 11% lower than in the placebo group.

In the Stockholm Ischaemic Heart Disease Study, nicotinic acid was used in combination with clofibrate. At five years there was a 26% reduction in total mortality and a 36% reduction in ischaemic heart disease mortality (Carlson *et al.*, 1988).

Nicotinic acid was used in combination with other drugs in several angiograph trials, including the CLAS and FATS studies, with positive results, as detailed on p. 73.

Adverse effects

Adverse effects associated with nicotinic acid are many and various. Undoubtedly this is a drug that requires a clinician experienced in its use. Furthermore, very detailed clinical and biochemical monitoring is required.

Most patients will experience cutaneous flushing associated with a prickly feeling in the skin, which can be frightening if the patient is not forewarned. This was a frequent finding a few years ago when the virtues of nicotinic acid were extolled in a book written for the lay public. Unsuspecting individuals having purchased large tablets (0.5 g) of nicotinic acid from health food stores were startled and alarmed by faces the colour of a ripe strawberry. Tachyphylaxis to the flushing occurs rapidly and aspirin is useful in alleviating this symptom (as it is in prostaglandin-mediated flushing). Other skin reactions include pruritus, rash, dry skin and (rarely) acanthosis nigricans.

Gastrointestinal side-effects including abdominal pain (peptic ulceration may be reactivated) and nausea are quite common. More serious but rarer adverse effects include cardiac arrhythmias. In the Coronary Drug Project atrial fibrillation occurred in 4.7% of the nicotinic acid group compared with 2.9% in the placebo group (Coronary Drug Project Research Group, 1975).

Cystic maculopathy leading to loss of visual acuity was observed in 0.7% of patients taking nicotinic acid at high dose (3–6 g/day). This disorder regresses after the drug is discontinued. Rarely myopathy can occur, with increased CPK levels.

Metabolic abnormalities are quite commonly associated with nicotinic acid therapy. Elevated uric acid levels can occur but precipitation of an attack of gout is rare. Glucose tolerance is decreased and this is particularly important if nicotinic acid is used in NIDDM patients. Elevated liver enzymes occur in up to 5% of patients and hepatic failure has been reported.

Indications

Nicotinic acid is widely used in the United States, where its relative cheapness is an advantage. In other countries (including the UK) it is rarely used because of the adverse effects described above. Attempts have been made to produce nicotinic acid derivatives to improve acceptability. Acipimox, for instance, received a licence in the UK. However, at the recommended doses this compound was considerably less effective than nicotinic acid.

Lack of availability of large-strength tablets also hinders the use of nicotinic acid in some countries. Some specialist clinics have arranged with their hospital pharmacy to import larger-strength tablets or to manufacture their own.

Nicotinic acid is indicated in all types of lipid disorder, either alone or in conjunction with other drugs. For the reasons indicated above it is relatively contraindicated in diabetics and patients at risk of cardiac arrhythmia.

FIBRIC ACID DERIVATIVES

First reports of these compounds appeared in the early 1960s. A series of phenoxyisobutyric acids led to reduction in both cholesterol and triglyceride in experimental animals. Of these compounds, clofibrate (chlorophenoxyisobutyrate) was developed for clinical use. Since then clofibrate has had a chequered career and is now largely redundant. However, several other fibrates have been developed that are generally more effective with less adverse effects on the lithogenicity of bile and gallstone formation – this was clofibrate's major problem.

Although these compounds have been available for study for over 30 years, their mechanism of action at a molecular level is only just beginning to be identified.

The fibrates are perhaps the most heterogeneous class of lipid-modifying drugs and clinicians experienced in their use often try a second member of the class if the first-choice agent fails to achieve the desired effect in a particular patient.

It is disappointing that there are not more large, controlled clinical trials with hard CHD end-points which have employed fibrates. Fibrates would be prime agents to test the hypothesis that reduction of hypertriglyceridaemia and elevation of HDL cholesterol will reduce CHD risk. These trials are still awaited.

Mechanism of action

The major action of fibrate drugs is to reduce plasma triglycerides; hepatic triglyceride synthesis is reduced and peripheral clearance is enhanced. The effects on the liver are thought to be secondary to reduced lipolysis in adipose tissue, with consequent reduced free fatty acid flux to the liver. The enhanced triglyceride clearance is due to an increase in activity of the enzyme lipoprotein lipase.

There has been much debate as to whether the fibrates inhibit cholesterol synthesis. There are reports of inhibition of cholesterol synthesis in experimental animals but these studies have been criticized because of the non-physiological drug concentrations used. Furthermore, results obtained in animals may not be applicable to humans.

Kinetic studies of lipoprotein turnover point to an effect of fibrate drugs on LDL clearance, probably through effects on LDL structure. By decreasing VLDL triglyceride and consequently VLDL size, fibrates enhance the production of rapidly catabolized LDL. LDL produced from smaller VLDL particles are larger and less dense and are better ligands for the LDL receptor. When fibrates are used to treat isolated hypertriglyceridaemia, LDL concentrations can increase, albeit from previous low levels. However, this increase in LDL mass is accompanied by a change in LDL distribution to larger, more buoyant particles.

HDL cholesterol concentrations tend to rise with fibrate therapy. This increase appears to be due to increased synthetic rates of apoproteins A-I and A-II, the major protein constituents of HDL. HDL concentrations may also be increased secondary to the reduction in triglycerides, which would tend to reduce the action of cholesterol ester transfer protein.

Conflicting reports are present in the literature in relation to the effects of various fibrates on lipoprotein(a) concentrations. As discussed elsewhere, lipoprotein(a) concentrations are mainly genetically determined and there is considerable length and sequence polymorphism in the apoprotein(a) gene. This may lead to the discrepant results in the literature, as patients are not matched for these genetic determinants. It is fair to say that as yet there is no convincing evidence of a fibrate effect on lipoprotein(a).

Despite the fact that it is over 30 years since the fibrate drugs were discovered it is only recently that clues have emerged with regard to their action at a cellular level. It is highly likely that fibrates induce a receptor called peroxisome proliferator activated receptor (PPAR), which belongs to the steroid and vitamin nuclear-receptor superfamily. When the receptor is converted to its active form it is capable of dimerizing with the 9-*cis* retinoic acid receptor. This complex can bind to response elements in the genome called peroxisome proliferation response elements, leading to regulation of important genes including acyl-CoA oxidase and fatty acid binding protein.

These exciting preliminary findings need to be confirmed in human studies.

Pharmacology and clinical efficacy

The availability of different fibrates varies from country to country. In the UK there are five licensed for clinical use: the original drug clofibrate together with gemfibrozil, bezafibrate, ciprofibrate and fenofibrate. In the United States, on the other hand, fibrate availability is limited to clofibrate and gemfibrozil.

Clofibrate, rapidly absorbed after oral administration, is hydrolysed to clofibric acid (p-chlorophenoxyisobutyrate), the active compound, peak plasma concentrations occurring at 6 hours. The drug is highly (95–98%) protein bound and the elimination half-life ranges between 12 and 25 hours and rises to 29–88 hours in patients with renal dysfunction. Approximately 60% is converted to the glucuronide and it is mainly excreted in the urine.

Gemfibrozil, although considered a fibric acid derivative, is structurally dissimilar to the other members of the class as it lacks the parachloride group. It is well absorbed with peak plasma concentration at 1 to 2 hours. The elimination half-life is approximately $1\frac{1}{2}$ hours. Gemfibrozil is highly metabolized, the major metabolite being a benzoic acid derivative. Seventy per cent of the drug is excreted in the urine – less than 2% unchanged. The drug does not appear to accumulate in patients with abnormal renal function. As with clofibrate, gemfibrozil is highly (95%) protein bound.

Bezafibrate, first introduced in 1978, is a second-generation clofibrate derivative. It is rapidly and completely absorbed with maximum plasma concentration at about 2 hours. Approximately 50% of the drug is excreted unchanged, with 22% as a glucuronide metabolite and 22% as unidentified metabolites. After 24 hours about 9% of the drug is excreted in the urine – the elimination half life being 2.1 hours. Bezafibrate is highly ($\simeq 94$–96%) protein bound.

Ciprofibrate is characterized by a long elimination half-life (80 hours) which enables once-daily dosing. Similar to other fibrates, it is rapidly and almost fully absorbed and the maximum plasma concentration occurs at 1 hour. There are three as yet unidentified metabolites but these constitute only a tiny proportion of the excreted dose. Seventy-three per cent of an oral dose is excreted in the urine as conjugated metabolites. The drug is highly (99%) protein bound.

Fenofibrate, first introduced in 1973, is rapidly and completely absorbed when taken with food. It is renally excreted and accumulates in patients with renal impairment. Fenofibrate is highly (99%) protein bound.

There are other fibric acid derivatives available for clinical use such as simfibrate, theofibrate and nicofibrate, and several others. As they are licensed only in a minority of countries (on average one or two) they will not be considered further here. Etofibrate, which is licensed in Spain, Germany and Switzerland, is the ethylene glycol diester of clofibric acid and nicotinic acid. After administration the drug is hydrolysed and the two active components are released. To date it does not appear to have any advantages over the usual fibrates.

The effect of fibrate therapy on plasma lipid and lipoprotein concentrations depends on the particular lipid phenotype and the particular fibrate chosen. As discussed above, there is considerable heterogeneity within the class, particularly with regard to effects on LDL cholesterol.

The major effects are on triglycerides and HDL cholesterol, as might be predicted from what is understood about their mode of action. The degree of triglyceride reduction is generally similar amongst the newer fibrates and depends on the baseline plasma triglyceride concentration. With high baseline levels, reductions of 60% would be expected.

Effects on LDL cholesterol of the various fibrates have been reviewed and on average gemfibrozil would be expected to produce a 10% reduction, bezafibrate a 15% reduction and fenofibrate and ciprofibrate a 25% reduction. As a general rule, LDL cholesterol reductions are greater in patients with pure hypercholesterolaemia than in those with mixed hyperlipidaemia. The paradoxical increase in LDL cholesterol in patients with hypertriglyceridaemia has already been discussed.

In addition to effects on plasma lipid levels various other potentially beneficial effects have been described with fibrate drugs. Fibrinogen, an important independent risk factor for CHD, is reduced by therapy with clofibrate particularly but also with bezafibrate, fenofibrate and ciprofibrate. Interestingly gemfibrozil does not appear to share this property. Other effects have been described on platelet function and other coagulation parameters but more studies are needed to clarify the situation. Gemfibrozil has been shown to decrease factor VII–phospholipid complex and plasminogen activator inhibitor-1 (PAI-1) activity, with consequent improved fibrinolytic capacity.

A frequent concomitant finding in hypertriglyceridaemic patients is hyperuricaemia and clinical gout. Fenofibrate therapy is associated with a sustained reduction in serum urate levels and this appears to be due to increased renal urate excretion.

Several major large, randomized, controlled clinical trials have assessed the effect of fibrate therapy on CHD events. In the Coronary Drug Project (see p. 183), 1103 middle-aged men with previous myocardial infarction received clofibrate for five years. Clofibrate therapy was associated with a modest 6% reduction in plasma cholesterol and a 16% reduction in plasma triglyceride. There was a reduction in fatal and non-fatal CHD in the clofibrate group compared with a placebo group ($n = 2789$) but this difference did not reach statistical significance. No difference in overall mortality was observed between the two groups.

In the large WHO Cooperative primary prevention trial (see p. 59), clofibrate (1.6 g/day) was given to approximately 5000 men whose cholesterol was in the upper third of the distribution. Individuals were followed for a mean of 5.3 years. Clofibrate therapy produced a modest 9% reduction in plasma cholesterol but this was associated with an overall decrease in CHD events of 20%, mainly due to a reduction in non-fatal myocardial infarction. However, deaths from non-cardiac causes were significantly higher in the treatment group. This finding, together with its limited efficacy and its undoubted predisposition to gallstone formation, has led to a decline in the use of clofibtrate and the drug is now virtually redundant.

In the Helsinki Heart Study (see p. 62), gemfibrozil (600 mg bd) or placebo was administrated to over 4000 middle-aged men with primary hyperlipidaemia (non-HDL cholesterol greater than 5.2 mmol/l). Gemfibrozil therapy reduced LDL cholesterol by 11%, plasma triglyceride by 35% and increased HDL cholesterol by 11% The cumulative CHD end-points (fatal and non-fatal myocardial infarction) at 5 years were 27.3/1000 in the treated group compared with 41.4/1000 in the placebo group, representing a significant 34% reduction.

In this trial non-cardiac deaths were not increased and there was no significant increase in the rate of cholecystectomy. The beneficial effects observed with gemfibrozil were related not only to the reduction in LDL but also to the increase in HDL cholesterol. In a subsequent analysis a subgroup with an LDL/HDL cholesterol ratio greater than 5 together with a triglyceride concentration greater than 2.3 mmol/l was identified as showing most benefit, with a 71% reduction in CHD events.

Further evidence on the potential benefits of fibrate therapy should emerge from current ongoing studies. The Bezafibrate Infarction Prevention (BIP) Trial is a secondary prevention trial being performed in Israel and gemfibrozil is the therapeutic agent in the High-density-lipoprotein Intervention Trial (HIT) being performed in the United States. Fenofibrate is the therapeutic agent in an angiographic regression study and also in a very large primary prevention trial in NIDDM patients coordinated from Australia (the FIELD Study).

Adverse effects

The fibrates are well tolerated in the majority of patients and adverse effects are infrequent. In some patients gastrointestinal symptoms (abdominal pain, diarrhoea and nausea) lead to discontinuation of therapy. Skin rash may occur very rarely. The most important side effect, which fortunately is rare, is myositis with muscle pain and tenderness and an elevated creatine phosphokinase level.

Fibrates tend to accumulate in patients with renal impairment, with the potential for increased side-effects – particularly myositis and deteriorating renal function. It is our practice to avoid the use of these drugs in such patients. Because the fibrates are highly protein bound they have the potential to potentiate the action of anticoagulants and careful monitoring is required.

There is no doubt that the founder drug, clofibrate, increases the lithogenicity of bile with resultant increased risk of gallstone formation. However, this problem is considerably less with later compounds. Cholecystectomy rate was not significantly increased in the Helsinki Heart Study and no excess gallstone risk has been reported with fenofibrate, which has the longest clinical experience after clofibrate. Biliary lipid studies in patients receiving ciprofibrate showed an increase in the cholesterol saturation in the short term but at one year there was no significant effect. It is sensible to avoid the use of fibrate drugs in patients with known biliary disease but the risk of gallstone development in those free of disease appears to be small. Occasionally elevations of liver enzymes are seen. However, alkaline phosphatase levels tend to be reduced consistently.

In rodents all fibrates produce hepatomegaly and peroxisome proliferation. This is species specific and does not occur in humans. Furthermore, hepatocellular carcinoma has been observed in rats receiving high dose fibrate therapy. Again this effect appears to be species specific. Nevertheless these findings, together with the increase in non-cardiac deaths observed in the WHO clofibrate trial, led to concerns on the long-term safety of the fibrate class. A recent meta-analysis of the fibrate trials has also cast doubt on safety, but the increase in non-cardiac mortality associated with fibrate therapy in the meta-analysis was entirely attributable to the data from the WHO study. It certainly appears that the newer fibrates should be viewed separately in terms of their safety from clofibrate. Certainly an interim safety statement from the long-term BIP study of bezafibrate did not give cause for concern.

Indications

Fibrates are first-line agents in patients with type III dyslipidaemia and in the treatment of moderate to severe hypertriglyceridaemia, and in mixed hyperlipidaemia where the predominant abnormality is hypertriglyceridaemia. They are not first-line agents for isolated hypercholesterolaemia.

Fibrates may be used in combination with anion exchange resins in mixed hyperlipidaemia and with nicotinic acid in severe hypertriglyceridaemia. In patients considered at high risk of CHD and mixed hyperlipidaemia, a fibrate may be used with a statin. Careful safety monitoring is required, because of the increased risk of side effects, and patients should be warned to stop the drugs in the event of muscle pains.

The considerable heterogeneity amongst the fibrate class has already been discussed. In our experience and based on published trials it is reasonable to infer that bezafibrate, ciprofibrate and fenofibrate are most effective in patients with isolated hypercholesterolaemia. In terms of triglyceride-lowering efficacy there seems to be little to choose between the drugs in mixed lipaemia. Gemfibrozil is particularly effective in type III dyslipid-aemia. In isolated moderate hypertriglyceridaemia, ciprofibrate and feno-fibrate are highly effective, whilst in the type V phenotype bezafibrate and gemfibrozil are most effective.

HYDROXY METHYLGLUTARYL COENZYME A (HMG COA) REDUCTASE INHIBITORS

The HMG CoA reductase inhibitors, sometimes referred to as the statins or, better, the vastatins, represent the newest class of lipid-lowering drugs to be introduced. They are inhibitors of cholesterol synthesis. Unlike earlier compounds such as triparanol and AY-9944, which inhibited steps towards the end of the pathway, resulting in accumulation of sterol-intermediates and resultant toxicity (cataracts, ichthyosis), the statins inhibit cholesterol synthesis at an early stage.

The first compound, compactin, was isolated from culture broths of the fungi *Penicillium citrinum* and *Penicillium brevecompactum*. This compound was not developed for clinical use and it was the structural analogues lovastatin and simvastatin, from *Aspergillus terrens*, and pravastatin (first identified as a urinary metabolite of compactin) that were eventually licensed. More recently, three synthetic analogs of the early fungal metabo-lites have been developed and brought to market in several countries: fluvastatin, atorvastatin and cerivastatin. The three compounds share a fluorophenyl group and a dihydroxyheptanoic side chain and atorvastatin has a polysubstituted pyrole nucleus (Figure 9.1).

Mechanism of action

These drugs are specific, competitive inhibitors of the enzyme HMG CoA reductase, which catalyses the rate-determining and first committed step in cholesterol synthesis – the conversion of HMG CoA reductase to mevalo-nate. The pathway is inhibited *in vivo* by approximately 40% as assessed by measurement of mevalonate concentrations. HMG CoA reductase enzyme protein increases when its activity is blocked but this does not overcome the inhibition.

As a result of inhibition of cholesterol synthesis in the liver, the prime target of the statins, hepatic LDL receptor activity increases, leading to

Figure 9.1
HMG CoA reductase inhibitors.

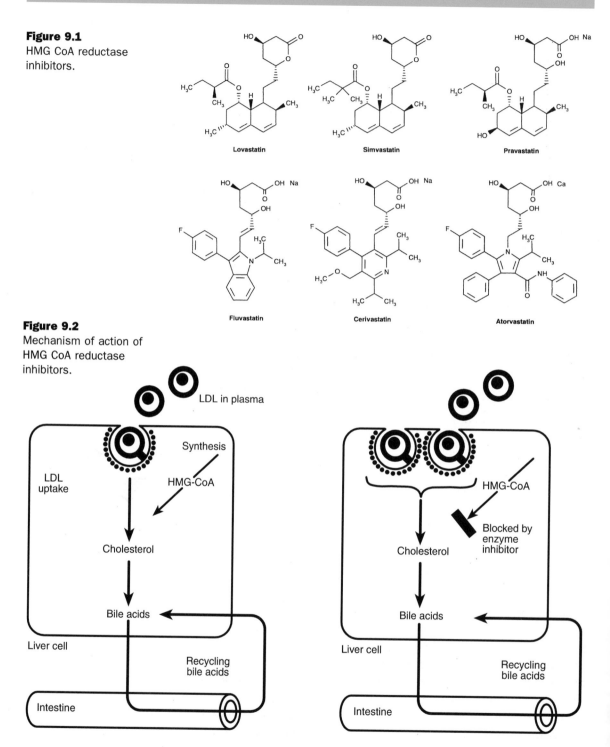

Lovastatin

Simvastatin

Pravastatin

Fluvastatin

Cerivastatin

Atorvastatin

Figure 9.2
Mechanism of action of HMG CoA reductase inhibitors.

LDL in plasma

Synthesis

HMG-CoA

LDL uptake

Cholesterol

Bile acids

Liver cell

Recycling bile acids

Intestine

HMG-CoA

Blocked by enzyme inhibitor

Cholesterol

Bile acids

Liver cell

Recycling bile acids

Intestine

increased uptake of LDL and decreased plasma LDL cholesterol and apoprotein B concentrations (Figure 9.2). In addition LDL cholesterol synthesis is decreased in some patients. That the statins principally act through the LDL receptor has been confirmed *in vivo* by lipoprotein turnover studies and *ex vitro* measurement of LDL receptor activity in liver biopsy specimens. As might be expected the statin drugs are much less effective in patients with homozygous familial hypercholesterolaemia. However, experimental high-dose simvastatin (86–160 mg/day) and atorvastatin have been shown to reduce LDL cholesterol significantly in these patients. It is likely, therefore, that in addition to effects on the LDL receptor there is also a reduction in hepatic VLDL output and consequently LDL production. VLDL synthesis is a complex process involving coupling of lipid (triglyceride and cholesterol) to apoprotein B facilitated by microsomal transfer protein. Inhibition of HMG-CoA reductase may affect this process and therefore reduce VLDL synthesis and output. This is also the probable explanation for the significant reduction in triglycerides.

Pharmacology and clinical efficacy

The statin drugs differ in the form in which they are administered: lovastatin and simvastatin are given as lactones, which are hydrolysed in the liver to the open acid form; pravastatin and fluvastatin, cerivastatin and atorvastatin, on the other hand, are administered in the open acid form. As can be seen in Figure 9.1, there is a striking structural similarity between the open acid parts of the statin molecule and the substrate, for the enzyme HMG CoA.

The absorption of statin compounds varies between the members of the class. Simvastatin, fluvastatin and cerivastatin are well absorbed (70–100%) and lovastatin ($\simeq$ 30%) and pravastatin ($\simeq$ 34%) less so. The degree of protein binding also varies: simvastatin, lovastatin, fluvastatin and cerivastatin are highly protein bound (> 90%) whilst pravastatin and its major metabolite show protein binding ranging between 46 and 57%. The elimination half-time of the statins is generally short (< 2 hours) and the major route of excretion is the liver. The elimination half-time of atorvastatin is longer (> 12 hours).

Much has been made in the past of the differences between the various statins with regard to lactone versus open acid form and the degree of solubility in aqueous or lipid environment, i.e. hydrophilic versus hydrophobic. Because of its free hydroxyl group at position 6 of the decalin ring (Figure 9.3), pravastatin is a hydrophilic compound whereas lovastatin and simvastatin are hydrophobic compounds as a result of the methyl group at this position. Fluvastatin is relatively hydrophilic. The differences in solubility characteristics may affect the degree to which the various drugs are taken up by non-hepatic tissues (hepatic uptake appears to be an active

Figure 9.3
LDL-C reduction by various HMG CoA reductase inhibitors (Black, 1994). *Recently, fluvastatin has been used and licensed at 80 mg/day dose which reduces LDL cholesterol by 31% (Schult and Beil, 1996). †Recently, data has been published on the effects of simvastatin at doses of 80 mg and 160 mg/day with reductions of LDL cholesterol of 47% and 53%. These doses are not yet approved (Davidson *et al.*, 1997).

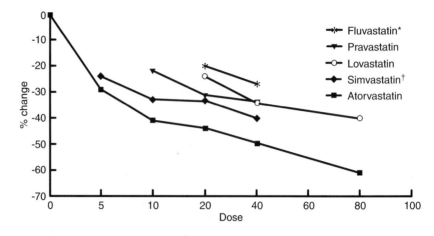

process) as hydrophobic compounds are better able to cross all membranes.

These differences, although undoubtedly present, do not appear to translate into significantly different clinical and biochemical adverse effects between the drugs. Through active uptake by the liver and major first pass metabolism and the degree of protein binding, the exposure of extrahepatic tissues to these compounds is very low.

The statins are the most potent compounds for reducing plasma LDL cholesterol concentrations. The efficacy and safety of the more established drugs have been reviewed (Illingworth and Tobert, 1994) and it is clear that simvastatin is the most potent of them. Furthermore, there is little evidence of significant safety issues between the various statins. Apoprotein B concentrations tend to be reduced to a similar degree as LDL cholesterol. HDL cholesterol concentrations tend to increase but only to a small degree ($\approx 5\%$), while triglycerides similarly show modest reductions (10–15%). Even more marked effects on plasma lipid and lipoprotein concentrations have been observed with atorvastatin. Reductions in mean LDL cholesterol of 60% have been observed with a dose of 80 mg/day administered to hypercholesterolaemic patients (Nawrocki *et al.*, 1995). In hypertriglyceridaemia patients, triglyceride concentrations fell by 25–43%. Atorvastatin also reduces LDL cholesterol ($\approx 30\%$) in homozygous FH patients. Cerivastatin is characterized by a much higher affinity for HMG-CoA reductase and high inhibitory activity allowing microgram dosage. At a dose of 300 μg, LDL cholesterol is reduced by 31%.

Statins have been studied in a wide range of patients. They appear to be effective in patients with type III disease, with significant reductions in LDL and VLDL remnants. They have been studied in patients with secondary dyslipidaemia, including diabetes and nephrotic syndrome, and beneficial effects on plasma lipid and lipoprotein profiles have been observed.

In severe hypercholesterolaemia, statins have been combined effectively with anion exchange resins, resulting in reductions of LDL cholesterol of approximately 50%. In severe mixed dyslipidaemia, statins have been combined with fibrates, with beneficial effects but careful safety monitoring is required with this combination as the risk of side effects, particularly myopathy, is increased (Shepherd, 1995).

Some of the statins have been used in long-term, randomized, controlled clinical trials to examine the impact of cholesterol lowering on hard CHD end-points. These trials have for the most part ended previous controversies in relation to adverse events. The landmark 4S study (p. 77) demonstrated a highly significant reduction in overall mortality in patients ($n = 4444$) with established CHD and cholesterol levels ranging between 5.8 and 8.0 mmol/l after dietary measures. A meta-analysis of trials performed with pravastatin in individuals with evidence of atherosclerosis ($n = 1891$) showed a highly significant reduction in CHD events and a trend to reduction in all-cause mortality which did not reach significance because of the low numbers. Various statins – lovastatin, pravastatin and simvastatin – have been used in many atherosclerosis regression trials either alone or in combination with other drugs. These trials (described in detail in Chapter 3) have shown that coronary plaque progression can be delayed and in some cases plaque regression can occur.

The first primary prevention trial using a statin was the West of Scotland study reported in 1995. This study showed that pravastatin therapy (40 mg/day) in middle-aged men with cholesterol concentrations of 6.5–8.0 mmol/l was associated with a highly significant reduction in the major study end-point of combined non-fatal myocardial infarction and cardiac death. No excess of non-cardiac death was observed such that overall mortality was also reduced.

Recently, LDL cholesterol reduction with diet and lovastatin has been shown to reduce ischaemic ST segment depression on ambulatory ECG monitoring in patients with proven coronary artery disease (Andrews *et al.*, 1997).

Adverse effects

With such potent drugs as the statins it is remarkable that the safety profile is so good. Generally the drugs are well tolerated and adverse effects leading to discontinuation of drug are rare.

The nature of their mechanism of action raised the possibility of adverse effects through inhibition of synthesis of important biological compounds – uniquinones and dolichols, formed from mevalonate. As can be seen in Figure 9.4, the biochemical pathways leading to ubiquinone and dolichol branch from farnesyl pyrophosphate prior to squalene synthetase. It is possible that inhibition of HMG CoA reductase could reduce flux through

Figure 9.4
Cholesterol synthetic
pathway showing the
branching points to
ubiquinones and dolichols.

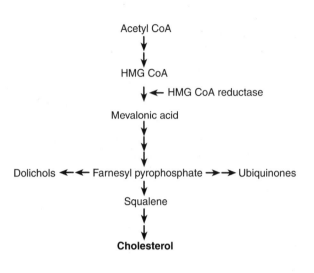

these pathways. Dolichol is required for glycoprotein synthesis and ubiquinone is important in mitochondrial electron transport. There does not appear to be any significant reduction in the synthesis of these compounds. As previously discussed, mevalonate levels are reduced by only 40% *in vivo* and the branch pathways appear to be preserved preferentially.

A further potential problem secondary to the action of statins is reduced hormone synthesis. Steroid hormones are produced from cholesterol and it is conceivable that reduction in cholesterol synthesis could be associated with a fall in adrenal and gonadal steroids. However, clinically significant reductions of steroid hormones have not been observed with statin treatment.

A further possible adverse effect which could be related to inhibition of cholesterol synthesis is reduction of bile acid synthesis. This could lead to an increased risk of gallstones through an alteration in the lithogenic index of bile. Bile acid production is probably moderately decreased by statin therapy, as shown by cholesterol balance studies. However, biliary cholesterol is reduced to a greater extent than bile acid production such that the lithogenic index is actually reduced.

The most common side effects of the statins are gastrointestinal disturbances but these tend to disappear if the drug is continued. Weakness, headache and aches and pains occasionally occur. Early studies in experimental animals given extremely high doses of some statin drugs had shown cataract formation. This has not been shown in human patients and ophthalmic assessment advised in early guidelines is no longer necessary.

The most serious adverse event with statin therapy is myopathy. This fortunately very rare complication is characterized by painful, tender muscles, often with 'flu-like symptoms. The creatine phosphokinase level is very high. Myopathy usually resolves when the drug is discontinued. In rare cases acute renotubular necrosis has occurred. Patients should be warned to stop statin drugs if they develop severe muscle pains.

Myopathy is more likely to occur when statins and fibrates are combined. Drugs that interfere with excretion of the statins, such as cyclosporine, nicotinic acid and erythromycin, resulting in raised blood levels, also increase the risk of myopathy. Statins are also best discontinued in severe intercurrent illness to avoid risk of myopathy, and should not be taken by individuals with liver dysfunction or by alcoholics.

Apart from the drugs discussed above, the potential for interaction of statins with other compounds is low. Statins do not appear to influence the cytochrome P450 system. The high protein binding of most of the statins should be remembered in patients who require anticoagulants. With pravastatin, however, no changes in anticoagulant action of warfarin have been observed.

Guidelines for biochemical safety monitoring during statin therapy have changed with increasing clinical experience. When the drugs were first introduced, frequent measurement of liver function tests was advised. This is not now necessary and it is our practice to check liver function prior to initiation of therapy and thereafter when the lipid profile is measured.

It is not our practice to measure creatine phosphokinase (CPK) levels routinely. Levels of this enzyme vary, often quite markedly, in normal individuals. However, if patients complain of muscle pain then it is important to measure CPK levels. An important practice point which is not generally known is the higher upper limit of normal for CPK levels in black patients.

Indications

In the United Kingdom, simvastatin (10–40 mg daily), pravastatin (10–40 mg daily), fluvastatin (10–80 mg daily), atorvastatin (10–80 mg daily) and cerivastatin (100–300 μg daily) are available for clinical use. In the United States lovastatin (10–80 mg daily), the first statin, is available, as it is in many other countries world-wide.

Statins are first-line agents for the treatment of hypercholesterolaemic patients in whom dietary and lifestyle measures have failed to achieve goals of therapy. They are also first-line agents in mixed hyperlipidaemia when the major lipid abnormality is raised cholesterol. In severe hypercholesterolaemia, such as heterozygous familial hypercholesterolaemia, statins can be used in combination with resins.

Combination of statins with fibrates is justified in severe mixed hyperlipidaemia in those patients considered to be at high risk of a coronary event. Increased safety monitoring is advised and intensive therapy of this nature is best left to the lipid expert. Similarly, in transplant patients receiving cyclosporine, careful monitoring is required in a specialized centre.

If statins are prescribed to premenopausal women of child-bearing potential, the patient should be counselled to discontinue therapy at least six weeks prior to planned conception.

Radical therapy for refractory hyperlipidaemia

Various forms of radical treatment have been used in patients with very severe hypercholesterolaemia, usually homozygous FH. These techniques are very much the province of the specialist centre.

ILEAL BYPASS

Prior to the advent of the statin drugs the treatment of heterozygous FH was unsatisfactory, particularly in patients who were unable to take large doses of anion exchange resins. This led to the introduction of partial ileal bypass by Buchwald in the United States (Buchwald, 1964). This operation involved sectioning the ileum and anastomosing it to the caecum so that the terminal third ($\simeq 200$ cm) of the ileum was bypassed. As a result the enterohepatic circulation was disrupted, with consequent increased hepatic bile acid synthesis and up-regulation of the LDL receptor just as with resin therapy. This operation was highly successful in reducing cholesterol levels and improved long-term outcome in terms of reduction of CHD, as demonstrated in the POSCH study (p. 75). Although post-operative diarrhoea was an occasional problem with this operation, it lacked the serious side effects of the jejunal ileal bypass used for obesity. As vitamin B_{12} is also absorbed from the terminal ileum, replacement vitamin B_{12} is required.

This operation is now largely redundant as most patients are tolerant of statin drug therapy. However, in the rare FH patient intolerance of all drugs then ileal bypass may still be indicated.

PORTACAVAL SHUNT

This operation has been used to treat homozygous FH – the rationale being to reduce hepatic lipoprotein production (Starzl *et al.*, 1983). Unfortunately the overall reduction in LDL cholesterol in two reported series was modest, ranging between 18% and 34%, and rarely was the total cholesterol reduced below 12 mmol/l. Xanthomata regressed in some patients but unfortunately most still succumbed to CHD. This operation is now redundant with the advent of liver transplantation and LDL apheresis.

LIVER TRANSPLANTATION

The first liver graft to a patient with homozygous FH was performed in 1984 in the United States (Starzl *et al.*, 1984). This operation will provide normal LDL receptors. The first patient was a 7-year-old girl who had already developed significant CHD requiring a heart transplant. Following this dual transplantation procedure her plasma cholesterol fell from 25 mmol/l to 7 mmol/l. There was a further cholesterol reduction with the statin drug, indicating that the LDL receptors on the transplanted liver were functional. Since then other homozygous FH patients have received this treatment, including a patient in the UK (Barbir *et al.*, 1992). Liver transplantation remains a high risk procedure and is reserved for FH homozygous patients who also require heart transplantation.

EXTRACORPOREAL LIPOPROTEIN REMOVAL

Various techniques have been developed for the regular removal of LDL from the circulation in patients with severe heterozygous or homozygous FH. These range from plasma exchange (Thompson *et al.*, 1975) to the more selective LDL apheresis, which employs the principle of affinity chromatography for the removal of apoprotein B-containing lipoproteins, leaving HDL to return to the patient (Richter *et al.*, 1993).

Using these techniques it is possible to produce substantial reductions in LDL cholesterol. For instance, twice-weekly sessions where 1–1.5 plasma volumes are passed through LDL apheresis columns results in a 40–50% reduction in integrated mean LDL cholesterol concentrations.

In the long term these techniques have been shown to lead to xanthomata regression, improvement in coronary atherosclerotic plaques and prolongation of life. However, these techniques are very expensive and can only be performed in specialist centres.

Another technique that has been used in Europe is the HELP system (Heparin Extracorporeal LDL Precipitation). LDL is precipitated from plasma by lowering the pH. The resulting precipitate is removed by filters;

the plasma pH is readjusted and returned. This process also removes fibrinogen and lipoprotein(a) (Thiery and Seidel, 1993).

GENE THERAPY

Homozygous FH is a prime candidate disease for trials of gene therapy, as current treatment options are relatively unsuccessful and the prognosis is very poor. A protocol is in place for gene transfer in the United States but current techniques are relatively crude, involving partial hepatectomy, the transfection of liver cells *ex vivo* with retrovirus carrying DNA for the LDL receptor and subsequent injection of the cells into the portal vein. The reduction in LDL in the first patient was relatively modest at 17% (Grossman *et al.*, 1994). Clearly gene transfer techniques are continually advancing and it is hoped that better results will be obtained in the future.

Part Four

Practical Considerations and Special Areas

The lipid clinic

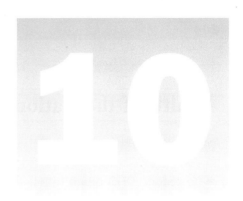

Running a lipid clinic in primary care

The term 'lipid clinic' is perhaps misleading as it tends to imply that the sole function of the clinic is to influence serum lipids rather than pursue a multifactorial approach to CHD prevention. It does, however, emphasize the central role of lipids in the genesis of CHD.

The importance of the need for CHD reduction ensures a prime role for primary care lipid clinics in health promotion programmes. GPs in the UK are now asked to design their own health promotion programmes relevant to the needs of their individual practices and localities as well as the themes of the Health of the Nation initiative. Through the primary care lipid clinic, specific high risk groups of patients can be offered integrated care – not only those with hyperlipidaemia, but also those with hypertension, diabetes and obesity, smokers and, above all, those with pre-existing coronary disease.

The primary care lipid clinic does not have to be a formal stand-alone clinic (cf. the antenatal clinic) but can be incorporated seamlessly into everyday practice as part of an integrated programme (in the same way that antenatal patients can be seen individually in normal surgeries). There is also considerable scope for a multidisciplinary approach involving other primary care team members.

To ensure that different team members impart the same health messages, it is helpful to establish agreed guidelines or, more formally, a practice protocol. Drawn from the available evidence this can form the basis of standard setting and can facilitate activity audit. For example, how many diabetics/hypertensives have undergone cholesterol measurement or how many patients with CHD are receiving lipid-lowering drugs? An example of locally produced guidelines is included below.

COMMENTARY ON THE GUIDELINES

The illustrated primary care guidelines are an example of locally produced guidelines influenced by the recommendations of the European

Health of the Nation targets for CHD

MAIN TARGETS

- To reduce CHD death rates:

  - in people under 65 by 40%
  - in people 65–74 years by 30%
  (by the year 2000 (compared with 1990).

RISK FACTOR TARGETS

- To reduce the prevalence of cigarette smoking in men and women over 16 to 20% by the year 2000 (1990 prevalence, 31% and 28%).
- To reduce the average percentage of food energy derived from total fat to 35% by 2005 (1990, 40%).
- To reduce the average percentage of food energy derived from saturated fatty acids to 11% by 2005 (1990, 17%).
- To reduce the percentage of men and women aged 16–64 who are obese (BMI > 30 kg/m^2) to 6% and 8%, respectively, by 2005 (1986/87, 8% and 12%).
- To reduce mean systolic blood pressure in the adult population by at least 5 mm Hg by 2005 (1991, 138 mm Hg)
- To reduce the proportion of men drinking more than 21 units of alcohol per week and women drinking more than 14 units per week to 18% and 7% by 2005 (1990, 28% and 11%).

Source: Department of Health (1993) *The Health of the Nation. A Strategy for Health in England*, HMSO, London.
Equivalent strategy documents exist for Wales, Scotland and Ireland.

Atherosclerosis Society and the British Hyperlipidaemia Association. They adopt a flow chart design from screening and result interpretation, through diagnosis and assessment, to interpretation and follow-up. All aspects are covered in greater detail in the wider context of this book.

Patients can be identified opportunistically, by systematic screening (see p. 85) or from disease registers (e.g. to identify patients for secondary prevention).

At initial interview, a decision about **whom to test** can be made using the selective screening list to identify those patients who may be offered cholesterol testing. A history or symptoms of CHD, PVD (peripheral vascular disease) or CVD (cerebrovascular disease) are elicited and an

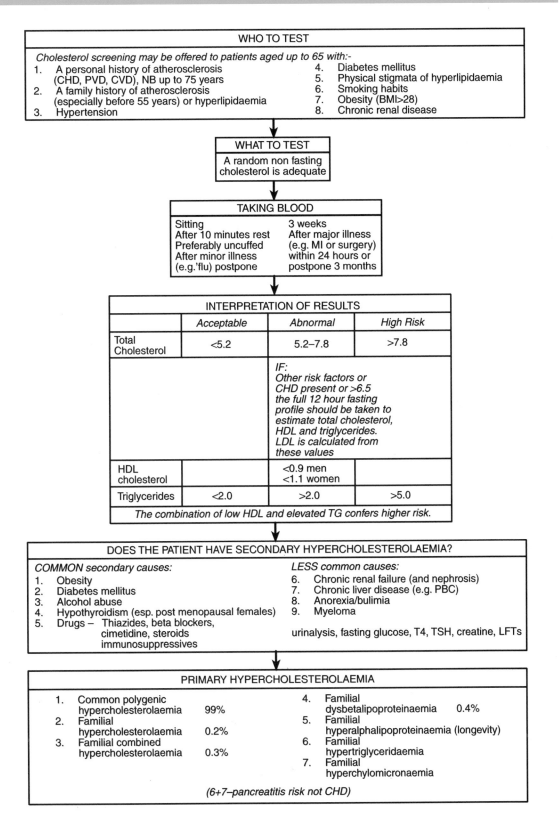

WHO TO TEST

Cholesterol screening may be offered to patients aged up to 65 with:-

1. A personal history of atherosclerosis (CHD, PVD, CVD), NB up to 75 years
2. A family history of atherosclerosis (especially before 55 years) or hyperlipidaemia
3. Hypertension
4. Diabetes mellitus
5. Physical stigmata of hyperlipidaemia
6. Smoking habits
7. Obesity (BMI>28)
8. Chronic renal disease

WHAT TO TEST

A random non fasting cholesterol is adequate

TAKING BLOOD

Sitting
After 10 minutes rest
Preferably uncuffed
After minor illness
(e.g.'flu) postpone

3 weeks
After major illness
(e.g. MI or surgery)
within 24 hours or
postpone 3 months

INTERPRETATION OF RESULTS

	Acceptable	*Abnormal*	*High Risk*
Total Cholesterol	<5.2	5.2–7.8	>7.8
		IF: *Other risk factors or* *CHD present or >6.5* *the full 12 hour fasting* *profile should be taken to* *estimate total cholesterol,* *HDL and triglycerides.* *LDL is calculated from* *these values*	
HDL cholesterol		<0.9 men <1.1 women	
Triglycerides	<2.0	>2.0	>5.0
The combination of low HDL and elevated TG confers higher risk.			

DOES THE PATIENT HAVE SECONDARY HYPERCHOLESTEROLAEMIA?

COMMON secondary causes:

1. Obesity
2. Diabetes mellitus
3. Alcohol abuse
4. Hypothyroidism (esp. post menopausal females)
5. Drugs – Thiazides, beta blockers, cimetidine, steroids immunosuppressives

LESS common causes:

6. Chronic renal failure (and nephrosis)
7. Chronic liver disease (e.g. PBC)
8. Anorexia/bulimia
9. Myeloma

urinalysis, fasting glucose, T4, TSH, creatine, LFTs

PRIMARY HYPERCHOLESTEROLAEMIA

1. Common polygenic hypercholesterolaemia   99%
2. Familial hypercholesterolaemia   0.2%
3. Familial combined hypercholesterolaemia   0.3%
4. Familial dysbetalipoproteinaemia   0.4%
5. Familial hyperalphalipoproteinaemia (longevity)
6. Familial hypertriglyceridaemia
7. Familial hyperchylomicronaemia

(6+7–pancreatitis risk not CHD)

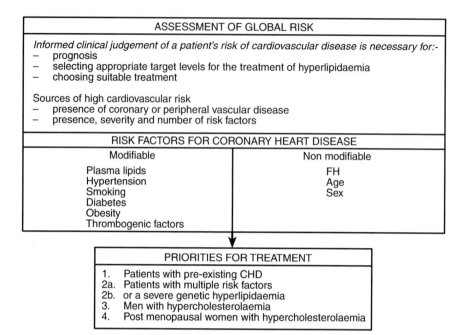

ASSESSMENT OF GLOBAL RISK

Informed clinical judgement of a patient's risk of cardiovascular disease is necessary for:-
– prognosis
– selecting appropriate target levels for the treatment of hyperlipidaemia
– choosing suitable treatment

Sources of high cardiovascular risk
– presence of coronary or peripheral vascular disease
– presence, severity and number of risk factors

RISK FACTORS FOR CORONARY HEART DISEASE

Modifiable	Non modifiable
Plasma lipids	FH
Hypertension	Age
Smoking	Sex
Diabetes	
Obesity	
Thrombogenic factors	

PRIORITIES FOR TREATMENT

1. Patients with pre-existing CHD
2a. Patients with multiple risk factors
2b. or a severe genetic hyperlipidaemia
3. Men with hypercholesterolaemia
4. Post menopausal women with hypercholesterolaemia

INTERVENTION

NON LIPID RISK FACTOR OPTIMISATION

Risk factor	Goal for treatment	Comments
Hypertension	Systolic BP < 160 Diastolic BP < 90	Treatment effective to 80 yrs but more difficult to achieve in the elderly. Thiazides and Beta Blockers may worsen co-existing hyperlipidaemia. Ca channel blockers and ACE inhibitors lipid neutral. Alpha blockers may improve lipid profiles. Beta blockers and ACE inhibitors to be used with caution in PVD.
Cigarette smoking	Cessation of smoking	Counselling and reinforcement may be required
Diabetes mellitus	Optimisation of lipids, BP, weight and glucose tolerance	More aggressive lipid and BP targets together with good glycaemic control are required. Nicotinic acid may worsen glucose tolerance
Obesity	Reduction ideally to BMI 20-25	Central obesity worse than peripheral
Family history of CHD	Unmodifiable	Useful in defining risk in proband and target family screening
Age	Unmodifiable	Value of lipid lowering therapy now proven to 75 years in secondary prevention
Sex	Unmodifiable	Premenopausal women relatively protected; consider hormone replacement therapy in post-menopausal women

DIET

Cornerstone of lipid lowering management. Cholesterol lowering diet with or without weight reducing diet. Maximises benefit of drugs if prescribed. Ideally individual consultation with dietician

DRUGS			
Drug	Side effects	Interactions	Comments
1. Hypercholesterolaemia (raised LDL)			
Bile Acid Sequestrants (RESINS) (colestipol, cholestyramine)	GI symptoms	Can prevent GI absorption of other drugs eg digoxin, thyroxine, anticoagulants, Fe, folic acid	GI side effects less likely, if introduced slowly. Most effective with or just before food. May increase TG. Give ather drugs 1 hr before or 4-6 hrs after.
HMG – CoA Reductase Inhibitors (STATINS) (atorvastatin, cerivastatin, fluvastatin, pravastatin, simvastatin)	GI symptoms Occasionally myositis and liver damage	Risk of myositis increased by fibrates, nicotinic acid and cyclosporine and erythromycin. Simvastatin and atorvastatin alter levels of anticoagulants and digoxin.	Best taken after food at night. Check LFTS regularly, CK if indicated.
2. Mixed Hyperlipidaemia (raised LDL + TG)			
FIBRATES (gemfibrozil, bezafibrate fenofibrate, ciprofibrate)	GI symptoms rarely myositis impotence	Anticoagulants 'Statins"	Best taken after food Increase HDL. Reduce TG
NICOTINIC ACID DRUGS (nicotinic acid, acipimox, nicofuranose)	Flushes and pruritis GI symptoms rarely liver damage and rashes		Aspirin alleviates, may worsen diabetes, gout and peptic ulcer
STATINS			Atorvastatin reduces TG by -20%
3. Hypertriglyceridaemia Fibrates and nicotinic acid drugs. omega 3 fatty acids (Maxepa)	GI symptons		
Safe combinations include resins with statins or fibrates.			

TARGET LEVELS FOR CHOLESTEROL AND LDL		
Global Risk	Reduce Cholesterol To	Reduce LDL To
MILD RISK e.g. TC 5.2 – 7.8 no non lipid risk factors	5.0 – 6.0	4.0 – 4.5
MODERATE RISK e.g. TC 5.2 – 7.8 plus 1 non lipid risk factor or plus HDL < 1.0	5.0	3.5 – 4.0
HIGH RISK e.g. CHD/PVD or TC > 7.8 or Familial Syndrome or TC 5.2 – 7.8 plus 2 non lipid risk factors or TC 5.2 – 7.8 plus 1 severe non lipid risk factor	4.5 – 5.0	3.0 – 3.5

FOLLOW UP	REFERRAL
4-6 weekly until target levels achieved and stable for two consecutive visits. Once stable monitor lipids (and where appropriate CK/AST/GGT) every 6-12 months.	Consider referral with – severe hyperlipidaemia (TC >9.0 or, TG > 5.0) – Familial syndromes – Established atherosclerosis with high lipids – Failure of initial drug therapy

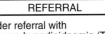

	SPECIAL SITUATIONS
Women	*Lipid risk assessment levels increased in premenopausal women by 0.5 – 1.0 mmol/L Women often have higher levels of HDL cholesterol which may also reduce risk. Consider HRT in postmenopausal women.* *Low fat diet safe in pregnant hyperlipidaemics. Lipid lowering drugs generally contra-indicated in pregnancy although bile acid sequestrants may be used on occasion; restart drug therapy postpartum after breast feeding completed; such patients are best monitored in hospital lipid clinics.*
Children	*Screening can be undertaken early in genetic hyperlipidaemias. Balanced low fat diet has been shown to be safe beyond age 5 yrs. Increasing use of drug therapy including statins. Such patients are best monitored in hospital lipid clinics.*
Elderly (> 65 years)	*Value of primary screening for hyperlipidaemia in patients over 65 yrs is unproven; those with established CHD, CVD and PVD, should be considered for intervention.*
Targeting patients with CHD	*All patients with MI should be targeted for screening and hypolipidaemic intervention either within hospital (<24 hrs) or at 3 months. Families of patients with MI under 55 yrs should be screened. Patients with angina, post CABG or angioplasty have been much neglected.*

enquiry made into family history and other risk factors for CHD. Lipid stigmata can be identified and baseline measurements of height, weight and blood pressure taken and recorded.

As the statin studies prove the benefit of cholesterol lowering in patients up to the age of 75, the age criteria can be extended to 75 in the secondary prevention situation.

In most instances, a random non-fasting cholesterol is adequate for **what to test**. There may be situations, however (for example, in secondary prevention), where there is an advantage in having as much information as possible and a fasting profile may be preferred.

Taking blood is a reminder of the need to standardize phlebotomy conditions and of the effect of intercurrent illness.

Repeated testing is required before management decisions can be taken, reflecting the biological and laboratory variation that cholesterol estimation suffers from and this is covered in **Interpretation of results**.

Patients without other risk factors and with serum cholesterol levels less than 5.2 mmol/l can be reassured but should be screened again in five years. LDL levels are calculated using the Friedewald formula:

$$LDL = \text{total cholesterol} - HDL - (\text{triglyceride}/2.19)$$

where triglyceride concentration is below 4.5 mmol/l.

Other causes of hypercholesterolaemia are excluded by asking the question: **Does the patient have secondary hypercholesterolaemia?** and an attempt at diagnosing **primary hypercholesterolaemia** can be made. In most cases the diagnosis will be the 'essential hypercholesterolaemia' of lipidology: common polygenic hypercholesterolaemia.

SCREENING
All adults 15–80
Case finding in primary care
3–5 yearly if normal

MEASUREMENT	
• Use standard mercury sphygmomanometer appropriately maintained and zeroed	• Take consistent measurements using the same arm, supported in the sitting position and without constricting clothing
• Use an appropriately sized cuff (within the 'range finder' narkers)	• Measure systolic BP and phase 5 diastolic BP (disappearance of sounds)– phase 4 (muffling) if no disappearance
Major sources of error include:	
Equipment faults	Observer faults
• mercury column not zeroed	• technique (eg not using Phase V sounds)
• leaking tubing/valves	• terminal digit preference (record to nearest 2 mm)
• inappropriate cuff size	• bias
Record 2 readings at each visit	
Level of readings will determine need for intervention. No intervention is made without repeated readings on different occasions. Standing pressures must also be measured in the elderly and diabetics (orthostatic changes)	
In AF take average of 3 readings; in subclavian stenosis take the arm with higher pressures.	
Repeated readings in identical circumstances may help eliminate 'White Coat Hypertension'	

INFLUENCES ON INTERVENTION

COEXISTING RISK FACTORS
Age > 60 years
Male sex
Hyperlipideamia
Smoking
Diabetes mellitus
Family history of cardiovascular disease

TARGET ORGAN DAMAGE
CHD – myocardial infarction, angina
Left ventricular hypertrophy
CVA/TIA
Renal impairment
Peripheral vascular disease
Retinal arterial changes

THRESHOLDS FOR INTERVENTION

DIASTOLIC BLOOD PRESSURE mmHg

Follow up	Severe ≥ 110	Moderate 100–109	Mild 90–99
At 1 W	≥ 110		Despite increased risk of CVA and MI potential benefit of pharmacological intervention more controversial
At 2 W	≥ 110 ↓ Treat	100–109 ↓ Treat if target organ damage	
At 1–2 m		100–109	90–99
At 3–6 m		100–109 ↓ Treat	90–99 ↓ Treat if 1. Target organ damage 2. Higher pressure in the range 3. > 60 years 4. Coexisting risk factors Observe the rest

SYSTOLIC BLOOD PRESSURE ≥ 160 mmHg

Treat if
- Target organ damage
- Remains raised after repeated measurements (over 6–12 months)

Isolated systolic hypertension less common < 60 years.
As yet no trial data on the potential benefits of treatment – recommendations based on extrapolation from elderly trial data.

SUMMARY

BP	Younger patients	Elderly patients > 60
DBP ≥ 100	Treat	Treat
DBP 90 – 99	Dependent on additional factors	Treat
SBP > 160	Treat	Treat

PATIENT INVESTIGATION

CLINICAL EXAMINATION

General appearance
Pulses (inc R-F delay)
Cardiac apex
Heart sounds (and signs of failure)
Renal mass / Bruit
CNS - evidence of CVA
Optic fundi
    (retinopathy grades 1–4)

SPECIAL INVESTIGATIONS

Urinalysis
Urea and electrolytes
Creatinine
Lipid profile (to 65 years)
Glucose
FBC (to detect raised MCV and polycythaemia)
ECG (?ECHO) for CHD/LVH

CXR may help in older patients

TREATMENT

NON PHARMACOLOGICAL TREATMENT

The Treatment Of Mild Hypertension Study showed that a combination of lifestyle changes could reduce BP by 10.5/ 8.2 mmHg. This may obviate the need for drugs, facilitate reduction using lower doses or avoid multiple drug combinations. All hypertensives should be offered this advice.

BP LOWERING
1. Achieve ideal body weight BMI 20-25
2. Avoid excess alcohol
Men 21 units Women 14 units
3. Reduce salt intake
4. Regular physical exercise

CARDIOVASCULAR DISEASE PREVENTION
As for BP lowering, plus
1. Stop smoking - the benefits of never having smoked far outweigh BP lowering
2. Reduce saturated fat intake to be replaced by monosaturates and polyunsaturates with increased fish, fruit and vegetables.

TREATMENT GOALS

SBP to < 160 mmHg
DBP to < 90 mmHg

PHARMACOLOGICAL TREATMENT

DRUGS
1. Thiazide diuretics
2. Beta blockers
3. Calcium channel blockers
4. Angiotensin converting enzyme inhibitors
5. Alpha 1 blockers
6. Angiotensin 2 blockers

FACTORS AFFECTING THE SELECTION OF DRUGS
1. Presence or absence of contraindications
2. Side effects
3. Coexisting disease.

PHARMACOLOGICAL TREATMENT SHOULD THEREFORE BE 'TAILORED' TO EACH INDIVIDUAL PATIENT.

USE OF ANTI-HYPERTENSIVE DRUGS IN A PATIENT WITH A SECOND CONDITION					
Coexisting disease	Diuretic	Beta blocker	ACE inhibitor	Calcium channel blocker	Alpha-blocker
Diabetes	Care needed	Care needed	Yes	Yes	Yes
Gout	No	Yes	Yes	Yes	Yes
Dyslipidaemia	Care needed	Care needed	Yes	Yes	Yes
Ischaemic heart disease	Yes	Yes	Yes	Yes	Yes
Heart failure	Yes	No	Yes	Care needed	Yes
Asthma	Yes	No	Yes	Yes	Yes
Peripheral vascular disease	Yes	Care needed	Care needed	Yes	Yes
Renal artery stenosis	Yes	Yes	No	Yes	Yes

SIDE EFFECTS					
Common side effects	Diuretic	Beta blocker	ACE inhibitor	Calcium channel blocker	Alpha-blocker
Headache	-	-	-	+	-
Flushing	-	-	-	+	-
Dyspnoea	-	+	-	-	-
Lethargy	-	+	-	-	-
Impotence	+	+	-	-	-
Cough	-	-	+	-	-
Gout	+	-	-	-	-
Oedema	-	-	-	+	-
Postural hypotension	+	-	-	-	+
Cold hands and feet	-	+	-	-	-

If clinical factors determining choice are equal consider cost. Start with lowest recommended dose and increase if ineffective but well tolerated. If remains ineffective in mild hypertension changes to another agent otherwise consider adding a second or third drug from another pharmacological class.

DRUG COMBINATIONS
May be required in up to half of cases. Examples of logical combinations includes: Diuretic + Beta blocker   Beta blocker + Calcium channel blocker + ACE inhibitor   + Alpha blocker ACE inhibitor + calcium channel blocker

FOLLOW UP	REFERRAL
Depends on severity, stability, compliance. When stable, every 3–4 m monitor efficacy of Rx, side effects, quality of life, risk and lifestyle factors.	1. Malignant hypertension is an in patient emergency. 2. Secondary hypertension 3. Significant target organ damage 4. Refractory hypertension - difficult to treat, wide fluctuations, rapid onset, worsening despite treatment.

THE ELDERLY
Patients aged 60-80 benefit from treatment when SBP > 160 mmHg or DBP > 90 mmHg. Evidence of benefit in treating very old people is lacking but it may be unwise to stop drug treatment unless blood pressure is normal and close monitoring of the effects of stopping treatment is available. Low dose thiazide diuretics are preferred as several trials show reduction in coronary events as well as CVA.

STOPPING TREATMENT
Patients (usually with mild hypertension) whose BP is consistently within target range (eg DBP < 80) may have their drugs reduced with careful monitoring. In some cases drug treatment may be withdrawn albeit subsequent regular long term monitoring and non pharmacological treatment are mandatory.

Having established that a patient is dyslipidaemic, an attempt must be made to assess the overall risk of CHD by **Assessment of global risk**. This is based on the well-known **Risk factors for coronary heart disease**.

The final step before intervention entails a consideration of which patients comprise **Priorities for treatment**.

Intervention involves **Non-lipid risk factor optimization** and **Diet** for all. Dietary management is pursued for as long as it continues to reduce lipid fractions towards **Target levels for cholesterol and LDL** and typically this may be from three to six months. Diet sheets abound but the personal approach of a health professional with nutrition skills is more effective. Inevitably not all high risk patients will achieve their target levels and consideration must be given to the addition of **Drugs**.

If drugs are prescribed, suggestions for monitoring their effects are included in **Follow-up**. Not all patients are straightforward and **Referral** lists some situations where the hospital clinic may be helpful.

Throughout the programme it is important to contain the patient's anxiety, to explain problems, negotiate and outline time limits in which to achieve realistic objectives. Accurate record keeping is required and several specific record cards are available. Computerization of records facilitates audit.

The communication of results should be effective and a call/recall system as employed in cervical cancer screening could be devised to eliminate defaulters and facilitate appropriate follow-up and rescreening.

Health checks in primary care

The discovery by Keys in his seminal Seven Countries Study (p. 26) that eastern districts of Finland had very high rates of CHD led to the foundation of a community-based project in North Karelia to target CHD. Since 1968 the rate of CHD has fallen more sharply in North Karelia than for the rest of Finland and the intervention programme has been hailed as a great success. In the Minnesota Heart Health Program (1986) a single exposure to an intensive educational component resulted in measurable life style and risk change. As recently as 1996, impressive changes in cardiovascular risk factors have been described by another community project in Mauritius.

In the UK in 1982, the Oxford Prevention of Heart Attack and Stroke project was initiated by Fullard, Fowler and Gray. A systematic approach by nurses greatly improved the recording of cardiovascular risk factors compared with opportunistic activity by GPs. The 1990 contract for UK GPs favoured health promotion activity for the first time and nurse involvement running 'Oxcheck' well-person and new-patient medicals was financially rewarded. Later a banding system was introduced allowing opportunistic as well as clinic activities. Doubts remained, however, about the efficacy of the checks in relation to health gain and a study in Powys, Wales (1993), suggested that well-person clinics were ineffective.

In 1994 the results (Table 10.1) of two large randomized, controlled, nurse-led screening and intervention programmes were published:

1. **Oxcheck Trial** (Muir, 1995) Participants aged 35–64 years were drawn from the patients of five group practices in three towns in Bedfordshire, England. After a 45-minute initial interview, the patients were followed up one year and three years later.
2. **British Family Heart Study** (Wood, 1994) In the BFHS, lifestyle screening and advice were given to men and their partners from 26 practices across 13 towns. Each town had a control practice as well as the

Table 10.1

Oxcheck Trial and British Family Heart Study (BFHS): summary of results (1994)

Risk factor	Reduction in risk factors (%) Oxcheck		
	Year 1	Year 3	BFHS
Total cholesterol	2.3	3.1 (♀ > ♂)	4.0
Systolic BP	2.5	1.9	7.0
Diastolic BP	2.4	1.9	
Smoking	0	0	5.0
BMI	0	1.4	
Diet	Improved (not significant)	Improved (significant)	
Dundee risk score			16

intervention practice. The interviews were longer and more intensive and the results were compared at one year.

Much publicity surrounded the publication of the results, which were considered disappointing considering the effort and the level of motivation of the researchers and the high expectations of benefit. However, when examined in terms of CHD risk reduction, Oxcheck showed a reduction of 6% in males and 13% in females due to cholesterol alone. The drop in BP over time could be an 'acclimatization' effect (noted in other studies) but if significant would further reduce CHD risk by 7%. The BFHS researchers calculated a 12% CHD risk reduction in men and almost the same in women. Small but significant benefits are thus evident. It is interesting to note that the results are comparable to the one year results of the North Karelia project, which eventually demonstrated a 40% CHD reduction over 20 years.

Cost-effectiveness data were published in the *British Medical Journal* in 1996 by Langham *et al.* and Wonderling *et al.*. In terms of life years gained, the more intensive BFHS intervention was more effective but less cost effective than the Oxcheck trial. The Oxcheck programme is cost effective if the effect lasts five years but the effect must last for about 10 years if the extra cost associated with the BFHS is to be justified.

Both of these studies extended invitations randomly to screening candidates irrespective of their cardiovascular risk factor profiles. Undoubtedly targeting specifically those patients at high risk would prove more cost effective.

Role of the hospital lipid clinic

It is our view that the hospital lipid clinic of today is equivalent to the hypertension clinic of the 1970s. The management of hypertension was then largely hospital based. However, over the years more and more patients with blood pressure have been identified and managed solely within the primary care setting.

The current situation with regard to the lipid clinic will vary depending on the interest and expertise of primary care physicians. Many GPs prefer to refer patients to the lipid clinic for an opinion on the advisability of drug therapy if lifestyle measures have failed. Although this approach is entirely reasonable, with increasing publication of definitive trials decisions on drug therapy can be made in primary care by following guidelines built firmly on evidence-based medicine. This approach can be highly productive and is best brought about by locally agreed protocols leading to a shared-care approach.

It is likely that the treatment of the more severe familial cases will remain in the lipid clinic. This is appropriate as often more complex investigation is required which is only available in specialist centres. These cases often need the back-up of non-invasive cardiac monitoring such as exercise cardiograms and thallium tests together with liaison with specialist colleagues, particularly cardiologists and cardiac and vascular surgeons. Often combination therapy is required, which is associated with increased risk of adverse events, and detailed safety monitoring is often easier in the hospital setting.

The lipid clinic is often involved in the assessment of new therapeutic approaches to the treatment of dyslipidaemia. In addition it has access to the more radical forms of therapy, e.g. plasmapheresis for severe FH. The lipid clinic often has a facility (usually through a specialist nurse) for family tracing, which is an essential part of the management of familial dyslipid-aemia. In some areas this can be accomplished using specialized genetic techniques.

There is no doubt that in the future more lipid patients will be treated solely in primary care, just as hypertensives are. The lipid clinic will remain a referral centre for the more difficult cases, familial dyslipidaemias, patients intolerant of first-line drugs, those individuals requiring multiple drug therapy, children and individuals with complex multiple problems.

The lipid clinic is usually led by a general physician with a particular interest in lipids. Often the physician has other interests as well, usually in diabetes or gastroenterology and occasionally cardiology. This is because there has not been a recognized speciality of lipidology, but training in lipidology in the UK is now recognized as an appropriate subspeciality by the Royal College of Physicians Committee on Diabetes and Endocrinology. It is hoped that the cardiologists will follow suit. In some districts the lipid clinic is run jointly by the chemical pathologist and a general physician. Most clinics have expert dietetic advice available within the clinic together with specialist nurses who assist in education, family tracing and research. Some clinics run specialist children's clinics with the help of the paediatrician.

In the UK, many lipid clinic physicians are members of the British Hyperlipidaemia Association (BHA), which holds an annual scientific meeting together with other specialist and teaching meetings. The BHA has produced guidelines for the management of lipid disorders and specialist publications dealing with children and clinical trials, amongst others. It publishes a list of known clinics and the specialist techniques that are available in particular clinics. The BHA is hoping to expand its membership (currently about 400) to include interested primary care physicians and practice nurses. This will help to disseminate knowledge and ensure that all patients with dyslipidaemia are optimally treated.

Special areas

The patient with established CHD

These patients should be the top priority for assessment and intervention. If an individual practice does nothing else in the lipid field, let it at least get to grips with the CHD patients. Sadly, current evidence points to under-recording and uptake of secondary prevention with lipid-lowering therapy in both specialist cardiac centres and district general hospitals.

The recent ASPIRE study (Action on Secondary Prevention through Intervention to Reduce Events) organized by the British Cardiac Society during 1994 and 1995 examined the clinical notes of a large patient population (> 2400 males and females) who had undergone a revascularization procedure or suffered myocardial infarction (ASPIRE Steering Group, 1996). Around half the men and three-quarters of the women studied had total cholesterol concentrations greater than 6 mmol/l at least six months after myocardial infarction or intervention. Of the small minority of patients on lipid-lowering therapy (8%), over half were inadequately controlled according to the British Hyperlipidaemia Association guidelines. This compares unfavourably with other European countries and the USA.

The evidence of benefit of cholesterol lowering in the patient with CHD is overwhelming and compares well with other interventions (Table 11.1). Based on the 4S study, using simvastatin, it was necessary to treat six patients for five years to prevent one event (death, coronary event, coronary artery bypass graft, angioplasty or stroke) (4S Study Group, 1994).

All patients with established CHD should have their lipid status assessed. In practice it is important to be aware of the falsely low cholesterol levels that can occur immediately post-myocardial infarction. Similarly, cholesterol measured in the early post-operative period following coronary artery bypass grafting may give falsely low levels. For this reason the fasting lipid profile is best assessed at three months.

The aim of therapy is to reduce the total cholesterol below 5.2 mmol/l. We prefer to use LDL cholesterol as the therapeutic target with a goal of therapy < 2.6 mmol/l. Nutritional and life style advice should be provided

Table 11.1
Benefits of long-term strategies for prevention of CHD in post-myocardial infarction survivors (Adapted from Sivers, 1996)

(a) Events prevented per 1000 patient-years of treatment

Treatment/strategy	Deaths prevented	Non-fatal events prevented
Aspirin[a]	7 vascular deaths	9 non-fatal reinfarctions 3 non-fatal strokes
Beta-blocker[b]	21 deaths	21 reinfarctions
HMG CoA reductase inhibitor (simvastatin)[c]	7 deaths	11 revascularizations 12 non-fatal infarctions 3 strokes 4 congestive heart failures
Smoking cessation[d]	15 deaths	46 reinfarctions

(b) Number of patients who need to be treated for 5 years (NNT)

Treatment/strategy	Events prevented	NNT to prevent one event
Aspirin[a]	CHD death, stroke or infarction	12
HMG CoA reductase inhibitor (simvastatin)*	CHD death, coronary event, CABG/PTCA or stroke	6
ACE inhibitor for left ventricular dysfunction: SAVE study[d]	CHD death or hospitalization for heart failure	10
SOLVD study[d]	CHD death or hospitalization for heart failure	21
CABG[e] for left main stem disease	CHD death	6

[a] Antiplatelet Trialists' collaboration (1994) *BMJ* **308**: 81
[b] Norwegian Multicentre Study Group (1981) *NEJM* **304**: 801
[c] 4S Study (1994) *Lancet* **344**: 1383
[d] Young (1994) *Heart Lung Transplant* **13**: 2135
[e] Laupacis (1988) *NEJM* **318** 1728

as first-line therapy for those with moderate hypercholesterolaemia. The patient should be reassessed at three months and hypolipidaemic drugs prescribed if the goal of therapy has not been achieved. Statins are the drugs of choice and the dose should be titrated upwards (6–8 weeks) until the goal of therapy is achieved.

Some patients will be taking anticoagulants. This should be borne in mind when starting statin therapy because of the potential for drug interaction (Chapter 10). It is prudent to arrange more frequent anticoagulant assessment. However, the anticoagulant therapy is not usually long term (often three months) and in most individuals the instigation of statin therapy can be delayed until warfarin is stopped.

It is unlikely that practices will have many patients who have undergone cardiac transplantation. However, it is important to note that these patients, as with other transplant recipients, are generally receiving cyclosporine therapy. This drug reduces excretion of the statin drugs, leading to higher serum levels and the potential for increased side effects such as myopathy. For this reason, statin therapy, which has been shown to be beneficial in these patients, is used at low dosage.

Some patients with CHD may have acceptable cholesterol levels but raised triglyceride and a low HDL cholesterol. The evidence of benefit in treating these individuals remains to be proved and ongoing clinical trials will provide more information. The recent bezafibrate study in young male myocardial infarction survivors (Ericsson *et al.*, 1996). (Chapter 10), though relatively small, does suggest that the drug-treated group in which there was no significant change in LDL cholesterol, but decreases in triglyceride and increases in HDL, shows similar affects for atherosclerosis progression/regression as seen in the trials using statin drugs. Obviously more clinical trial information is required but it is our practice to treat individuals with raised triglycerides ($>$ 2.3 mmol/l) when associated with a low HDL cholesterol.

Children and adolescents

Early lesions of atherosclerosis have been described in post mortems of adolescents. From a public health perspective it would be a reasonable proposition to initiate prevention measures for CHD in childhood and adolescence, when dietary and exercise habits are developing. Furthermore, anti-smoking advice and education is imperative.

Severe genetic lipid disorders, such as familial hypercholesterolaemia and familial defective apoprotein B, which markedly increase CHD risk, are expressed from birth. In addition, familial combined hyperlipidaemia is identifiable in adolescents from affected families. Familial chylomicron-aemia syndrome may present in childhood, with risk of pancreatitis.

Approaches to screening children and adolescents for lipid disorders vary from country to country and there are marked differences between the two sides of the Atlantic. Recommendations from the US's National Cholesterol Education Program (NCEP) Expert Panel on Blood Cholesterol Levels in Children and Adolescents advocate a comprehensive screening strategy with LDL cholesterol cut-points for intervention with dietary and drug therapy (National Cholesterol Education Program, 1992). In the UK the practice has been a more selective approach designed to identify major inherited disorders of lipoprotein metabolism, particularly familial hypercholesterol-aemia.

The main recommendations of the NCEP panel are as follows.

- A lipid profile should be performed if parents or grandparents developed coronary atherosclerosis leading to need for intervention therapy below the age of 55 years.
- A lipid profile should be performed if parents or grandparents or aunts and uncles developed myocardial infarction, angina, peripheral vascular disease, cerebrovascular disease or sudden cardiac death below the age of 55 years.
- Screen for hypercholesterolaemia in offspring of a parent found to have a plasma cholesterol concentration greater than 240 mg/dl (6.5 mmol/l).
- When history is unavailable on parents or grandparents, children and adolescents who have two or more cardiovascular disease risk factors may be screened at the physician's discretion.

These screening measures may be performed after two years of age. The NCEP LDL cholesterol cut-points for children from high risk families are shown in Table 11.2.

The British Hyperlipidaemia Association's recommendations for screening for hyperlipidaemia in childhood (Neil *et al.*, 1996) can be summarized as follows.

- The principal aim of screening should be to identify children with FH.
- A selective screening strategy should be used.
- Selection should be based on a family history of FH or premature coronary disease.
- A non-fasting total cholesterol measurement is a suitable screening test.
- If the cholesterol concentration is above 5.5 mmol/l, fasting measurement of total cholesterol, HDL cholesterol and triglycerides is required.

(a) Cut-points for total and LDL cholesterol

Level	Total cholesterol		LDL cholesterol	
	mg/dl	mmol/l	mg/dl	mmol/l
High	≥ 200	5.2	30	3.4
Borderline high	170–199		110–129	
Acceptable	≤ 170	4.4	≤ 100	2.6

(b) Guidelines for use of drug therapy: children 10 years or older

Risk factors for vascular disease	Post-dietary LDL cholesterol	
	mg/dl	mmol/l
None	≥ 190	4.9
Positive family history for premature CHD or two or more other CHD risk factors	≥ 160	4.1

Table 11.2
National Cholesterol Education Program Expert Panel on blood cholesterol in children and adolescents (1992, *Paediatrics* **89** 525–584)

- The diagnosis of FH in a child under 16 years should be based on finding a total cholesterol concentration above 6.7 mmol/l and an LDL cholesterol concentration above 4.0 mmol/l and requires at least two measurements, to be made more than one month apart.
- Children should not usually be screened before the age of two years, but the aim should be to diagnose heterozygous FH before the age of 10 years.
- Affected children should be referred for specialist care.

Not surprisingly, we incline towards the UK view on screening in children, with the major emphasis on identifying FH. The mainstay of therapy in FH children is dietary. Low fat diets do appear to be safe, as long as sufficient calories are provided.

The use of hypolipidaemic drug therapy in children remains a matter of judgement for the specialist. The main factor that argues for drug therapy is early onset CHD in the family. If a first degree relative developed CHD in the third decade then drug therapy should be started after the age of 10 years. Girls with FH are less likely to require intervention with drugs unless there is premature CHD in a female relative. We also measure lipoprotein(a) as a further indicator of risk.

The drugs of choice are the anion exchange resins, which are not systemically absorbed. There has been no reported evidence of vitamin deficiencies, fat malabsorption or adverse effects on calcium or vitamin D metabolism. Folic acid levels decrease and supplements are advised. These drugs can cause problems with compliance, as they are tiresome to take, and in that event the HMG CoA reductase inhibitors may be considered. As a general rule, we do not start therapy with statins till late teenage. There are trials of statins in adolescents lasting two to three years and no significant changes in growth and development were observed.

In addition to diet and drug therapy for the hypercholesterolaemia, strong anti-smoking advice should be given together with general advice on a healthy life style, particularly the benefits of regular exercise. Children are best managed in a special clinic run in conjunction with a paediatrician.

Women and CHD

The discovery in the early American epidemiological studies of the increased prevalence of CHD in middle-aged men has led to the erroneous assumption that CHD is predominantly a male condition. The stereotypic victim of CHD remains, in the eyes of most people, the 45-year-old stressed businessman. For economic reasons, cardiovascular research, prevention and intervention have often been targeted at men and relatively few studies incorporate data on women. Even treatment recommendations arise by extrapolation from the data on men.

The presentation of the symptoms of CHD varies between the sexes. Women tend to present with angina more commonly than infarction and their symptoms are sometimes atypical. There is a bias towards non-cardiac diagnosis, especially in younger women. In addition the incidence of coronary artery spasm (Syndrome X) is increased and, as a result, exercise ECG testing is less reliable.

During the last five years there has been considerable debate concerning CHD in women, with accusations of misogyny and neglect being levelled at health professionals. Women suffer higher mortality after myocardial infarction and at the time of coronary artery revascularization and they attend less for cardiac rehabilitation. Whilst there is evidence for increased delay in reaching hospital and reduced thrombolysis rates, it may be that much of the difference between the sexes relates to the fact that presenting women are older, with more advanced disease in biologically smaller arteries.

Around the world the distribution of CHD in women closely mirrors that of men, with remarkably constant sex differences. In the UK the chance of dying from CHD before the age of 65 for a man is 3.5 times that for a woman, but after 65 the rates are more equal. As we have seen, women lag 7–10 years behind men in peak CHD incidence. With an ageing population, more female CDH deaths are to be expected. CHD has already become the commonest cause of death for women in the UK and the USA, responsible for one in four deaths, and in the USA CHD is now responsible for proportionately more deaths in women than men.

There have been many attempts to explain these differences and discussion has centred on:

- sex roles
- parity
- hormonal effects
- risk factors.

SEX ROLES

Gender stereotyping weakens the impact of sex roles and their contribution to CHD risk. For example, the innate aggressive, hostile, competitive, coronary-prone behaviour of men is contrasted with the compliant, supportive, nurturing behaviour of women. The assertion that leaving home to work imparts extra stress to men is disputed by every housewife and data exists showing reduced CHD in women who work away from home.

PARITY

Having more than five children is associated with an increased CHD risk of 20%. Possible causes discussed include lower socio-economic status, the effect of hormonal influences in pregnancy or the stress engendered by child-rearing. Data from the Rancho Bernado study in the United States, however, suggest that the effect is obesity mediated.

HORMONAL EFFECTS

Data from Framingham and the Nurses Health Study convincingly demonstrate that the risk of CHD in women is increased after the menopause. The fact that a hormonal effect (endogenous oestrogen) may be active had been suggested by Robinson in 1959 when women who had had a premature oophorectomy had been shown to suffer increased rates of CHD. It is important to remember, however, that CHD still occurs before the menopause; indeed, one in four CHD deaths in women under 65 years old occur before age 45. It is commonly supposed that LDL levels suddenly increase as the menopause occurs but Figure 2.10 shows that LDL starts to increase at about 30 years, increases steadily to 55 and then plateaus.

The attraction of the hormonal theory is further diminished by the lack of support from serial laboratory measurements of oestrogen for a protective effect.

RISK FACTORS FOR CHD IN WOMEN

The risk factors for CHD in women tend to be the same as for men but with quantitative differences in their effects. Women tend to have higher levels of blood pressure, cholesterol and fibrinogen and a greater incidence of diabetes but reduced central obesity and smoking levels and increased HDL (Figure 2.10).

Cholesterol

Whilst increasing cholesterol still relates to increasing CHD, total cholesterol (or LDL) becomes a much weaker predictor of CHD in women than in men. For example, in the Renfrew and Paisley study in the West of Scotland, the absolute risk of women 45–64 years old with cholesterol levels in excess of 7.2 mmol/l was still less than that in men with levels < 5.0 mmol/l. This is just as well, as by 55 years old in the UK one in three women have cholesterol levels exceeding 7.8 mmol/l.

HDL levels

Mean HDL levels tend to be higher in women throughout life compared with men and, because of the inverse relationship with CHD, HDL provides another popular explanation for the observed sex difference. That HDL cannot be the sole explanation is shown by the observation that when men and women with the same HDL levels are compared, women still fare better. Low HDL is a less powerful predictor of CHD risk compared with men but values < 1.1 mmol/l nevertheless are associated with increased risk. Ratios comparing total cholesterol or LDL to HDL can be useful in evaluating risk.

Triglycerides

Data from Framingham and Gothenburg both show the increased predictive potential of raised triglycerides for CHD and even suggest independence as a risk factor. When the relative strengths of different lipid risk factors are compared by likelihood ratio analyses, the order in women is HDL > triglycerides > LDL.

Obesity

As with cholesterol, the predictive capacity of obesity measured in terms of weight or BMI is reduced in women. The distribution of adipose tissue seems more important and measures of central obesity (e.g. WHR > 0.8) are more powerful predictors. As in men, the obesity itself contributes little to the increased risk of CHD but it is the relationship with associated risk factors such as diabetes, dyslipidaemia and hypertension that promotes the risk.

Hypertension and diabetes

Hypertension is a strong risk factor in women. Diabetes provides the greatest example of gender difference, the presence of diabetes completely neutralizing a woman's sex advantage in CHD risk.

Smoking

Although smoking levels are generally lower than in men, dose-dependent increased CHD risk is still evident in women. Smoking more than 40 cigarettes a day increases CHD risk 20-fold. There is concern at the levels of smoking in younger women who, already victims of social stresses and targeted advertising, may also smoke to control weight.

Oral contraceptives

Most early epidemiological studies found an increased risk of myocardial infarction in current users of the combined oral contraceptive pill. This was not unexpected, given the effect of ethinyl oestradiol on CHD risk markers, but reduction in dose and pharmaceutical reformulation together with avoidance of use in high risk groups have improved safety. Women taking a third-generation combined oral contraceptive such as low-dose ethinyl oestradiol plus gestodene or desogestrel are no more likely to have a myocardial infarction than non-pill takers. Preliminary data from recent studies, however, suggests that third-generation pill users are less likely than second-generation pill users to have a myocardial infarction, but this risk needs confirmation and is offset by an increased risk in venous thromboembolism. In the UK this has led to a change in prescribing practice in favour of older products. It is possible that third-generation pills were deliberately prescribed to women with other risk factors (age, smoking, obesity) to lessen their risk and that the change in recommendations is inappropriate.

The combined oral contraceptive pill does cause a significant rise in BP (mean 6/4 mm Hg) and this supports usual clinical practice to monitor patients at six-monthly intervals.

MENOPAUSE AND HORMONE REPLACEMENT THERAPY (HRT)

In 1994 Stampfer published a meta-analysis of observational studies which showed that post-menopausal hormone replacement therapy with oral oestrogen almost halved the risk of CHD. Most of this action seems to be mediated through lipoprotein mechanisms, though improved arterial function and insulin sensitivity are also suggested.

The effects of the menopause and oestrogen replacement therapy on lipoproteins are summarized in Figure 11.1. At the menopause there is an increase in total cholesterol, LDL (particularly of the small dense atherogenic variety), Lp(a) and triglyceride. HDL is slightly reduced but this

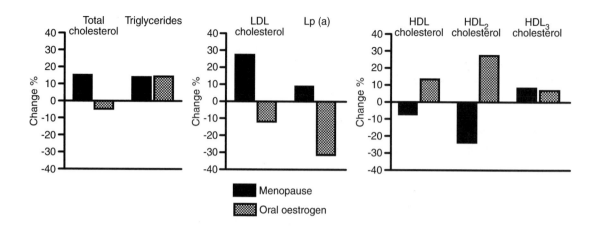

Figure 11.1
Effects of the menopause
and conjugated equine
oestrogen (0.625 mg) on
lipoproteins. Source:
Crook and Stevenson
(1996) *Lipids: Current
Perspectives*, p. 179,
using data from
Stevenson, Lobo and
Jenner.

disguises a large reduction in HDL2 with a slight rise in HDL3 and a consequent increase in CHD risk.

Adding oestrogen reverses these changes, producing a fall in total cholesterol and LDL (by 10–15%) and a rise in HDL (chiefly HDL2) and triglycerides. Progestogens are necessary for endometrial protection but androgenic progestogens, such as norethisterone and levonorgestrel commonly used in the UK, oppose the effect of oestrogens, raising LDL and reducing HDL. Medroxyprogesterone acetate is the leading progestogen used in the USA and its effect in combination with oestrogen is summarized as HDL ↑, LDL ↓, triglycerides slightly ↑, Lp(a) ↓, factor VII ↑, fibrinogen ↓. In addition, there are beneficial effects on glucose metabolism, antioxidant activity has been demonstrated *in vitro* and endothelially mediated effects promote coronary artery relaxation.

The prospect of reducing CHD in post-menopausal women by nearly 50% is tantalizing and would seem to suggest 'oestrogen for all'. Women who take HRT, however, tend to be a generally healthier cohort, better educated and of higher social class than women who do not. In addition, they are leaner in build, have increased medical supervision in follow-up and therefore are at lower CHD risk before the benefits of HRT are added. A large compliance bias may also produce a strong placebo effect. It will not be until the publication of randomized controlled trials such as the Heart Estrogen/Progestin Replacement Study (HERS) by the end of the decade and the National Institutes of Health investigation in 2008 that such issues will be resolved.

Trends in hormone replacement therapy

● **Transdermal delivery systems (patches)** Transdermal delivery negates the rise in triglycerides seen in oral replacement (which may be important for those with hypertriglyceridaemia) and even produces a reduction. Unfortunately the fall in LDL and rise in HDL are also reduced.

- **Continuous combined HRT** In an effort to minimize the nuisance of menstruation by continuous endometrial suppression, continuous combined regimes have been marketed. Unfortunately most use androgenic progestogens, which reduce HDL.
- **Tibolone** Again, Tibolone is marketed to avoid the need for menstruation. Whilst there is no effect on LDL concentrations, HDL is reduced by 20%.

Given the array of hormones and the ingenuity of the pharmaceutical industry, it should be possible to design the ideal preparation, the most likely candidate at present being an oestradiol/dydrogesterone combination. From a cardiovascular point of view, oral oestrogen remains the best answer and it is interesting to speculate whether more lives would be saved using oestrogen alone to prevent CHD than lost by abandoning endometrial protection with progestogens.

Considering HRT as treatment to reduce CHD risk

Apart from the treatment of climacteric symptoms and osteoporosis, there is a role for HRT in the reduction of CHD risk and this is acknowledged in recent guidelines such as ATP II (p. 140). In the presence of hypercholesterolaemia (> 8.0 mmol/l) plus other risk factors, HRT may confer benefit but the benefits are debatable in isolated hypercholestrolaemia.

LIPID LOWERING IN WOMEN

Early data suggest benefit in secondary prevention and genetic disorders such as FH. In the CARE study (Chapter 3) the risk reduction for major coronary events in women was more than double that for men (46% versus 20%).

The elderly patient

It is often asked whether therapy should be initiated in the elderly. This begs the question as to what age constitutes 'elderly'. The definition will change as the questioner grows older! As a general rule, in all decisions with regard to initiation of treatment strategies, attention should be focused on biological rather than chronological age.

Important issues to consider when addressing lipid-lowering therapy in the elderly are:

- the predictive value of lipoprotein concentrations in older age groups;
- the limited lifespan;
- concomitant morbidity with increased potential for adverse effects of drugs;
- potential adverse effects of dietary restrictions;
- paucity of trial evidence.

Although there is much epidemiological evidence linking total cholesterol, LDL cholesterol, HDL cholesterol and triglyceride to CHD risk in men and women over the age of 65 years, relationships may be less strong than in younger populations. However, as the burden of CHD increases with age, so the attributable risk increases, though the relative risk with increasing cholesterol levels diminishes. This important concept is demonstrated in Figure 11.2.

In some studies HDL cholesterol appears as a particularly important predictor in the elderly. In the 'very old', conflicting data exist. In a study from the USA – the Bronx Ageing Study of men and women aged 75–85 years – a low HDL cholesterol ($\leqslant 0.78$ mmol/l) was associated with increased CHD in men and a high LDL cholesterol (> 4.4 mmol/l) with CHD in women (Zimetbaum et al., 1992). In a further 4-year prospective study, no association was found between plasma cholesterol and CHD in individuals aged more than 70 years (mean age 79 years) (Krumholz et al., 1994).

In men and women with established CHD aged more than 65 years in the Framingham study, a high cholesterol (> 7.1 mmol/l was associated with an increase in recurrent disease four-fold higher than that observed with a low cholesterol (< 5.1 mmol/l) (Wong et al., 1991).

Most trials of lipid-lowering therapy on CHD end-points have been performed in middle-aged populations but men and women up to the age of 70 years were included in the 4S study. When the results were analysed

Figure 11.2

Risk for CHD mortality with age in the top cholesterol quartile (upper line) vs. bottom quartile (lower line). Shaded area is the attributable risk due to cholesterol, which can be seen to increase with age. Source: Rubin et al. (1990) Ann. Intern. Med. **113**, 916–920.

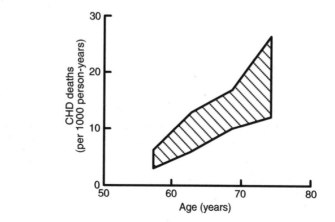

according to age, similar benefits of therapy were observed in those aged more than 60 years as in those below 60 years. Similarly, in the CARE study of pravastatin in secondary prevention, men and women were included up to the age of 75 years and benefit was observed in the older subgroups.

The results of these recent studies confirm those of an early Stockholm Secondary Prevention Study, which included patients up to 70 years of age. Drug therapy consisting of a combination of nicotinic acid and clofibrate was associated with a decrease in CHD and overall mortality, in those aged over 60 as well as those under 60 years.

On the basis of the above discussion it would seem appropriate to initiate lipid-lowering therapy in older individuals with clinically overt vascular disease. Both epidemiological and trial data support this. Furthermore the benefits of cholesterol reduction are seen early. More and more, the benefits of coronary artery bypass grafting are being made available to the older patient and it is our view that these individuals should receive therapy. The case for primary prevention in the elderly remains more difficult and more trial information is required. It is possible that, just as with hypertension therapy, benefits of cholesterol lowering would be observed.

The hypertensive patient

Hypertension is an important risk factor for atherosclerotic vascular disease. It has been known for many years that the major CHD risk factors interact to multiply risk. This is illustrated in Figure 11.3 with data taken from the Framingham study. It can be seen that the relative risk of CHD in relation to hypertension depends on both the concomitant LDL and HDL cholesterol concentration (Kannel, 1983).

Hypertension and dyslipidaemia commonly occur together in the same individual. Depending on the population studied and the definition adopted, the prevalence of hypercholesterolaemia in hypertensives ranges from 28 to 43% (MacMahon *et al.*, 1985). This is perhaps not surprising since dyslipidaemia and hypertension share common environmental determinants, such as obesity. Furthermore these factors are both components of the insulin resistance syndrome which no doubt involves the interplay of genetic and environmental factors, such as obesity and lack of physical activity. Williams and colleagues in Utah, USA, have described the familial association of essential hypertension and dyslipoproteinaemia in a study of 58 families. These authors have suggested that the association may occur in about 12% of hypertensives (Williams *et al.*, 1988).

Trials of anti-hypertensive therapy have demonstrated unequivocal benefit in terms of stroke reduction but the impact on CHD (which in quantitative terms is a much more significant cause of death and morbidity)

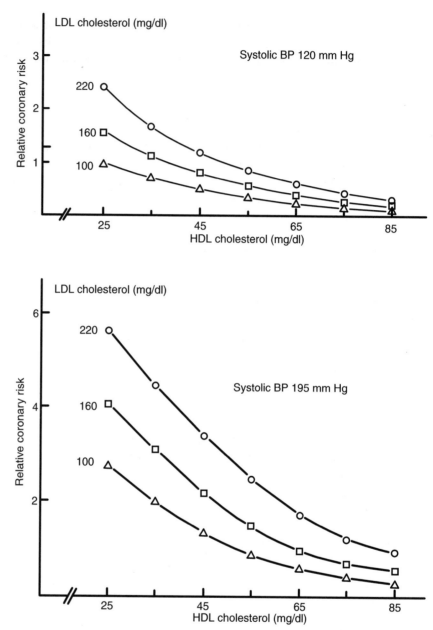

Figure 11.3
Relative coronary risk in relation to HDL cholesterol at different levels of LDL cholesterol in normotensive and hypertensive individuals. Source: Kannel (1983).

was less. Nevertheless, when the trials were combined in meta-analysis by Collins and colleagues, it was apparent that there was a reduction of 14% in total CHD (Collins *et al.*, 1990). This reduction is less than would be expected from the observational data linking hypertension to CHD risk.

The discrepancy between the observed and expected benefit of blood-pressure lowering on CHD has received much discussion. A possible contributing factor is the potential for adverse metabolic effects of anti-hypertensive agents used in the trials, particularly high dose thiazides and beta blockers (Krone and Müller-Wieland, 1990). In a cross-sectional study of hypertensives performed in Australia, the prevalence of dyslipidaemia was indeed higher in patients established on treatment compared with newly presenting untreated patients (MacMahon *et al.*, 1985).

There have been many trials of the effects of various anti-hypertensive agents on plasma lipid and lipoprotein concentrations (Krone and Müller-Wieland, 1990). A summary of these findings is shown in Table 11.3. It should be remembered that many of the studies used what are now recognized to be excessive doses, e.g. bendrofluazide 10 mg. It is likely that metabolic effects are minimal at low doses, e.g. bendrofluazide 2.5 mg. A further point to remember is that these studies were not performed in dyslipidaemic subjects. It is likely that anti-hypertensives with adverse metabolic effects will produce more marked changes where dyslipidaemia or glucose intolerance already exists. In fact it has been reported that the use of beta-blockers so exacerbated hypertriglyceridaemia as to precipitate pancreatitis.

The question arises as to whether dyslipidaemia should be treated in the hypertensive. CHD risk is multiplied when more than one risk factor is present, which argues for an aggressive policy towards concomitant dyslipidaemia with life style changes and, if necessary, hypolipidaemic drugs. Most middle-aged hypertensives will fulfil the risk criteria that make the use of hypolipidaemic therapy a practical and cost-effective intervention.

A further question is whether concomitant dyslipidaemia should influence the choice of anti-hypertensive agent. It is our opinion that it should. The approach to the patient at risk of CHD should address all modifiable risk factors and the epidemiological data suggest that even small changes in

Table 11.3

Effects of anti-hypertensive drugs on lipid and lipoprotein concentrations

Drugs	Total cholesterol	LDL-C	HDL-C	TG
α-Blockers	↓	↓	↑	↓
Vasodilators				
Calcium antagonists	→	→	→	→
ACE inhibitors				
Diuretics	↑	↑	→↓	↑
β-Blockers				
B$_1$- and non-selective	→	→	↓	↑
Intrinsic sympathomimetic activity	→	→	→↑	↑
Vasodilatory properties	→	→	→	→

cholesterol or HDL cholesterol may have important long-term effects on CHD risk. However, it should be remembered that the trials showing benefit of treatment of hypertension have been performed with beta blockers and thiazides. Comparative studies with newer classes of anti-hypertensive therapy are needed. In the meantime, if there are no specific indications for agents such as beta blockers (e.g. angina or post-myocardial infarction), our practice is to choose agents that do not have adverse metabolic effects.

The diabetic patient

Management of the diabetic patient offers substantial challenges for not just the restoration of well-being but also the prevention of long-term complications. The Diabetes Control and Complications Trial (DCCT) has demonstrated unequivocally that improved glycaemic control is associated with delayed onset and progression of retinopathy, neuropathy and nephropathy in insulin-dependent diabetics (IDDM) (Diabetes Control and Complications Trial Research Group, 1993). In our opinion these results are likely to be applicable to non-insulin-dependent diabetic (NIDDM) patients.

There have been significant advances in the treatment of diabetic nephropathy, particularly the appreciation of the need for careful blood pressure control and the protective effect of angiotensin-converting enzyme inhibitors. The use of laser therapy for the treatment of retinopathy has been a major factor in reducing visual loss from maculopathy and proliferative retinopathy.

Advances in the prevention and management of microvascular complications have not been accompanied by similar advances in what is the major cause of morbidity and mortality in diabetic patients, namely, large vessel disease. Atherosclerosis is more extensive and occurs at an earlier age such that CHD, stroke and amputation occur at an increased incidence.

In a cohort of IDDM patients followed up at the Joslin Diabetes Center in the USA, cumulative CHD mortality at the age of 55 years was about one-third, which represents a six-fold excess compared with a control population drawn from the Framingham study (Krowlewski *et al.*, 1989). In NIDDM patients there is a high prevalence of CHD at the time of diagnosis and CHD incidence is increased at least three-fold compared with age-matched and sex-matched controls (Kannel *et al.*, 1979; Margolis, 1973). Several studies have demonstrated the particularly high relative risk for diabetic women (Barrett-Connor and Wingard, 1983). Diabetic patients with established CHD have a poorer prognosis than non-diabetic CHD patients (Abbott *et al.*, 1988). It is increasingly recognized that proteinuria in diabetic patients is an extremely important predictor of risk for overall mortality and particularly CHD death (Borch-Johnsen and Kreiner, 1987). The mechanism of this relationship remains to be fully determined.

The recent St Vincent Declaration has called for a reduction in morbidity and mortality from CHD by vigorous programmes of major CHD risk factor reduction (Krans *et al.*, 1992).

Plasma cholesterol concentration is an important independent risk factor for atherosclerosis-related disease in diabetic patients, as it is in non-diabetics. This has been shown in many studies, including the massive database of the men ($n = 347\,978$; aged 35–57 years) screened for the Multiple Risk Factor Intervention Trial (MRFIT) (Stamler *et al.*, 1993). Cardiovascular death was increased three-fold in diabetics ($n = 5163$) independent of serum cholesterol, blood pressure and cigarette smoking, which confirms the independent association of diabetes with vascular risk. However, increasing cholesterol was associated with increased cardiovascular death rates in both diabetic and non-diabetic men and the absolute risk relationship was steeper in the diabetic group (Figure 11.4). This was also true for cigarette smoking and blood pressure and when the three risk factors were combined. From these findings the authors of this analysis of MRFIT argued for rigorous intervention to lower cholesterol, abolish cigarette smoking and control blood pressure in diabetics.

As might be expected, it is LDL cholesterol that correlates with the presence of vascular disease in diabetics, while HDL is inversely related to disease particularly in NIDDM patients. Plasma triglycerides also appear to be an important risk marker for vascular disease in diabetic patients.

Typical lipid abnormalities in IDDM patients (with and without nephropathy) and NIDDM patients are shown in Figure 11.5. It can be seen that total cholesterol concentrations are not different to controls except when

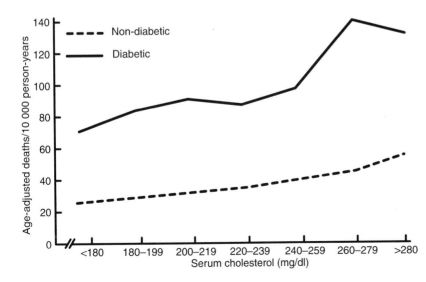

Figure 11.4
Diabetic and cardiovascular disease in MRFIT: CVD death rates by serum cholesterol (mg/dl). Source: Stamler *et al.* (1993)

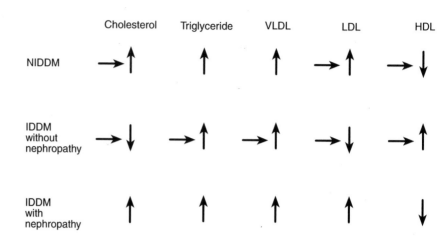

Figure 11.5
Quantitative lipid and lipoprotein abnormalities in diabetes mellitus, assuming reasonable glycaemic control.

glycaemic control is poor. Nevertheless the high risk of diabetes argues for aggressive management. Hypertriglyceridaemia, often associated with low HDL cholesterol, is the lipid hallmark of NIDDM and often persists in patients on established diabetic therapy. Those diabetics with nephropathy tend to have a higher prevalence of lipid disorders, which no doubt contributes to the increased risk but does not fully explain it.

It is likely that LDL cholesterol has increased atherogenic potential in diabetes because it is susceptible to glycation, which delays clearance from the circulation. It also appears to be more sensitive to oxidation. Furthermore, in the presence of hypertriglyceridaemia small dense LDL accumulates, which is more atherogenic.

Hypertriglyceridaemia in NIDDM patients is associated with accumulation of atherogenic remnant particles and abnormal postprandial lipaemia in addition to increased coagulation factors such as factor VII and the anti-fibrinolytic factor, plasminogen activator inhibitor I.

A full fasting lipid profile should be incorporated into the annual assessment of diabetic patients. Goals of therapy for lipid management in diabetics have been provided by the European Working Group (Alberti and Gries, 1988) on the management of NIDDM (Table 11.4) and the American Diabetes Association (Consensus Statement 1993). Other causes of secondary dyslipidaemia should be excluded, particularly hypothyroidism and renal disorders. The choice of anti-hypertensive agents in the diabetic should be exercised with care in view of the adverse effects of some agents on lipids. Primary dyslipidaemias should be treated as described elsewhere. It is unlikely that severe hypercholesterolaemia and hypertriglyceridaemia will be due solely to diabetes, and an underlying primary disorder exacerbated by diabetes is likely.

If attention to improved glycaemic control, diet and life style do not lead to satisfactory improvement of the lipid profile then a case can be made for

Targets for metabolic control	Good	Acceptable	Poor
Blood glucose (mmol/l)			
Fasting	4.4–6.7	< 7.8	> 7.8
Post-prandial	4.4–6.9	< 10	> 10
HbA$_1$	< Mean + 2SD	< Mean + 4SD	> Mean + 4SD
Urine glucose (%)	0	< 0.5	> 0.5
Total cholesterol (mmol/l)	< 5.2	< 6.5	> 6.5
HDL-cholesterol (mmol/l)	> 1.1	> 0.9	< 0.9
Fasting triglycerides (mmol/l)	< 1.7	< 2.2	> 2.2
Body mass index (kg/m^2)			
men	< 25	< 27	> 27
women	< 24	< 26	> 26

Table 11.4
Metabolic targets (Alberti. K.G.M.M. and Gries, F.A., 1988, *Diab. Med.*, **5**, 275–281

lipid-modifying drugs. The drugs of choice in diabetes are the statins and fibrates. Nicotinic acid and fish oils may exacerbate glycaemic control and resins may exacerbate hypertriglyceridaemia.

No CHD primary or secondary prevention trials of lipid-lowering drugs have been performed specifically in diabetic populations. A small group of diabetics was included in the Helsinki Heart Study but the numbers were insufficient to give significance, though a trend to benefit was observed (Koskiner *et al.*, 1992). Approximately 200 diabetics were included in the 4S secondary prevention study. When all cardiovascular end-points were pooled, a significant benefit was observed in the diabetics (Pyörälä *et al.*, 1995). Similar results have been found in the CARE study (Sacks *et al.*, 1996).

Other primary and secondary prevention trials are in progress in diabetics using statins (the atorvastatin CARDS study) and fibrates (the fenofibrate FIELD study). Until these trials report, it is reasonable to treat diabetics with established CHD along the lines of the 4S study and to take into account the high intrinsic risk of diabetes when deciding on primary prevention.

The patient with peripheral vascular disease

Patients with peripheral vascular disease have a four- to six-fold increase in risk of CHD. Peripheral vascular disease can be diagnosed on the basis of clinical signs and symptoms of ischaemia with abnormalities of ankle–

brachial pressure ratios or flow velocities. Many of these individuals will attend surgical clinics and it is likely that risk factor assessment is inadequate, particularly with regard to plasma lipids.

Why in some patients there should be a predisposition for peripheral vascular disease remains to be determined but prospective epidemiological and clinical studies point to the high frequency of underlying CHD in these cases. Peripheral vascular disease is a frequent occurrence in type III dyslipidaemia, which is associated with the accumulation of remnant lipoprotein particles. NIDDM patients also have a high risk of peripheral disease and similarly tend to accumulate remnant particles.

Patients with peripheral vascular disease deserve to be treated just as those with established CHD because of their high risk. It is of interest that an early randomized angiographic study (Duffield *et al.*, 1983) performed in patients with stable intermittent claudication demonstrated that lipid-lowering drug therapy was associated over a 19-month period with significantly fewer arterial segments which showed detectable progression. The mean increase in plaque area in the treatment group was only one-third of that in the untreated group. Furthermore, mean increase in the edge irregularity index (a measure of the severity of the disease) was 40% of that observed in the untreated group. There was a positive correlation between mean LDL cholesterol concentration achieved during the trial and the rate of disease progression ($r = 0.59$; $P < 0.05$).

The patient with cerebrovascular disease

Patients with significant carotid artery disease with clinical symptoms of transient ischaemic attack or stroke or identified by the presence of an arterial bruit with subsequent ultrasound or angiographic investigation are also at high risk of CHD.

Such individuals merit aggressive lipid-lowering therapy, as long as this is not militated against by advanced age or disability or deterioration in mental function. The goals of therapy should be those adopted for individuals with symptomatic CHD. Lipid-lowering therapy should complement aspirin treatment and careful attention should be paid to blood pressure control.

Recent lipid-lowering intervention trials using HMG CoA reductase inhibitors have demonstrated that progression of carotid atherosclerosis, as assessed by the intima-medial thickness, can be reduced. The effects appear to be confined largely to the common carotid with little effect being observed at the bifurcation or the internal carotid.

In the Kuopio Atherosclerosis Prevention Study (KAPS), pravastatin therapy was associated with 64% reduction in progression in the common carotid, but no effect was observed in the bifurcation (Salonen *et al.*, 1995). Similar results have been observed in the Pravastatin Lipids and Athero-sclerosis in the Carotid Arteries (PLAC-II) study (Crouse *et al.*, 1995) and in the Asymptomatic Carotid Atherosclerosis Plaque Study (ACAPS) (Furberg *et al.*, 1994) which employed lovastatin. In PLAC-II almost all the effect on carotid intima-medial thickness could be explained by the reduction of LDL cholesterol.

As discussed previously, an incidental but important finding in the three major statin end point trials (4S, CARE and WOSCOPS) was a reduction in the incidence of stroke which reached statistical significance.

Economic aspects

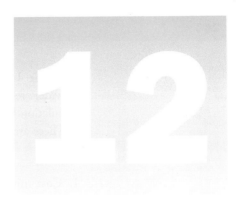

Each year in the UK, CHD costs an estimated £1 billion with a further £0.5 billion expended in benefit payments. In addition, the hidden cost to industry in lost production is estimated at £3 billion. In the United States, direct medical expenditure exceeds $100 billion.

Any initiatives to improve the health of individuals or a nation should be evidence based. This means that decisions should be based on the conclusions of randomized trial evidence and a consideration of the benefits and risks of the intervention against the pre-intervention prognosis. Unfortunately, as the number of health gain initiatives is potentially large and as resources are finite, new initiatives must also satisfy economic considerations. In future, cost-effectiveness parameters should be built into the design of all randomized controlled trials.

In the UK, 90% of health care is provided by the National Health Service with purchasers having an increasing influence on the provision of services by providers. In contrast to other countries the UK, with centrally cash-limited funds, has been able to control health care costs despite the pressures of an ageing population, expensive medical advances and increased demands from the population. The amount expended on health as a percentage of gross domestic product is considerably less than other westernized countries (Table 12.1) but it is debatable whether this represents efficiency or underprovision of care.

Table 12.1
Health care costs (1987)

County	% of GDP	£ per head
United States	11.2	1236
France	8.6	666
West Germany	8.0	658
Japan	6.9	551
UK	6.1	457

In the United States, health care providers dominate the purchaser/provider relationship but the system is undermined by 30% of the population being either uninsured or inadequately covered.

There are four main methods of economic evaluation:

1. **Cost minimization analysis** Here two interventions are compared only in terms of cost, the cheapest being the preferred option. No account is taken of differing effectiveness.
2. **Cost effectiveness analysis** Here costs are compared with units of outcome. For example, in a cholesterol management programme the costs of screening, testing, professional time, monitoring and treatment can be related to a 1 mmol/l drop in cholesterol for a hypercholesterolaemic individual. A more common comparison is the cost per life year gained.
3. **Cost–benefit analysis** This requires the benefits of an intervention to be valued in purely monetary terms. Consideration is given to the valuation of production gains or how much an individual would be willing to pay for the intervention. The analysis can be difficult to interpret.
4. **Cost–utility analysis** This is an extension of cost effectiveness and relates both the quantity and quality of life gained from a health care intervention. For example, a year of full quality life is one QALY (quality adjusted life year).

In 1990, Reckless examined the costs of a community cholesterol screening and treatment programme over 10 years for patients aged 20–64 years (Table 12.2). The overall QALY cost was £550 ($\male$ £370, $\female$ £1090). Where diet alone was employed the QALY cost was £120 and where drugs were needed (in 3.7% in this analysis), the QALY cost rose to £3060 ($\male$ £2080, $\female$ £6130). Apart from the predictable difference between the sexes, the QALY costs for the older age groups were less than the QALY costs for younger groups and this reflects the rising prevalence of CHD with age.

In the same year, the Standing Medical Advisory Committee (SMAC) in the UK published a similar analysis of the costs of a cholesterol management programme in the 40–69 age group. By including other risk factors the costs of QALYs were shown to reduce, the lowest costs relating to males with pre-existing CHD or multiple risk factors. Not surprisingly the patients at highest risk receive the most cost effective benefit.

The QALY costs for cholesterol lowering compare favourably with other health care interventions already well established in everyday practice.

Intervention	Cost per QALY (£)
Cholesterol management (community)	550
Cholesterol management (drugs)	3060
Coronary artery surgery (marked angina/main vessel disease)	1300
Coronary artery surgery (mild angina/single vessel disease)	15 300
Screening for breast cancer	5500
Screening for cervical cancer	5500

Table 12.2
Comparison of QALY costs for cholesterol lowering with established health care interventions

The QALY cost for haemodialysis has been estimated at £26 683 and this is an intervention that tends not to be denied patients in advanced health care systems.

Economic considerations of the Scandinavian Simvastatin Survival Study (4S)

The size and statistical power of this landmark study allow pharmaco-economic consideration of its implications (Reckless, 1996).

The cost of simvastatin in the 2221 patients in the active treatment group for 5.4 years with 90% compliance is approximately £6 million. For the 74 fewer deaths from all causes and 78 fewer CHD deaths, the cost per life saved works out at £80 900 for all-cause mortality and £76 800 for CHD mortality.

Although life expectancy tables by current age for Scandinavia are not yet available, the life expectancy of 4S participants is reduced anyway by virtue of their pre-existing CHD. Making certain assumptions, Reckless calculates the number of life years saved and cost becomes approximately £8200 per life year saved.

If the costs of the reduction in morbidity are then taken into account (191 fewer CHD events, 131 fewer coronary artery operations) and the benefits in terms of extra life years are added, the final benefit of simvastatin falls to around £3060 per life year saved. If estimates of improved quality of life were available, QALY cost would be yet more impressive.

Some of the prospectively collected data on the use of health resources for the 4S study have been presented. Admissions to hospital and operative procedures (CABG and angioplasty) are reduced by 32%. CVA rates are reduced by 30% and total days spent in hospital by 34%. A cost minimization analysis (Pedersen, 1996) using 4S data extrapolated to the United States, showed that 88% of the cost of simvastatin could be offset by the reduced number of hospital contacts. The effective cost of simvastatin works out at 28 cents/day, or 41 cents/day if the costs of laboratory monitoring are added. Jönsson *et al.* (1996) in a cost effectiveness analysis suggested a cost of £5500 per life year saved, and when indirect costs are taken into account this analysis even suggests cost savings in certain groups (for example, younger patients). These sums per life year saved are more cost effective than the treatment of mild hypertension and chronic renal failure.

Preliminary calculations following the publication of WOSCOPS (p. 64) have suggested that the cost of pravastatin treatment is $\leqslant$ £10, 000 per life year saved in men fulfilling the criteria of the primary prevention trial design. As patients with pre-existing CHD are more likely to have further events, it is no surprise that the cost effectiveness of secondary prevention is greater than that of primary prevention. The WOSCOPS investigators did not intend to suggest blanket treatment for all, but early subgroup analysis does not suggest that those with additional risk factors derive more benefit from cholesterol lowering. For example, smokers received similar benefit compared with non-smokers (see p. 65).

A different approach is taken by Pharoah and Hollingworth (1996) whereby the results of 4S and WOSCOPS are applied to a health authority population in the UK using life tables to estimate life years gained by statin therapy. In their model population of 500 000 there are 50 000 males aged 45–64 years. The cost effectiveness of primary prevention statin treatment is £136 000 per life year saved and for secondary prevention £32 000 per life year saved – potentially prohibitive expenditure for any health authority. These averages hide large variations in cost effectiveness; for example, for a male aged 45–54 with a history of MI and a cholesterol $>$ 7.2 mmol/l, the cost is £6000 per life year saved.

Drug	Daily dose	Cost (£)
Cholestyramine	24 g (6 sachets)	810
Colestipol	30 g (6 sachets)	915
Bezafibrate	400 mg	110
Ciprofibrate	100 mg	175
Fenofibrate	200 mg	320
Gemfibrozil	1200 mg	385
Fluvastatin	20–80 mg	195–390
Pravastatin	10–40 mg	210–605
Simvastatin	10–40 mg	240–610
Atorvastatin	10–80 mg	245–1225
Cerivastatin	100–300 µg	170–240

Table 12.3
Approximate costs of drugs for one year's treatment (1997 prices); Source: MIMS (Monthly Index of Medical Specialities), February 1997

There have been many criticisms of this analysis and the estimated input costs of the study were considerably higher than those calculated by Reckless. True cost-effectiveness figures will not be available until both costs and life years gained are accurately established.

Few medical treatments have received the intensity of cost speculation accorded to lipid lowering therapy – and this is appropriate, given the scale of the problem and the potential for benefit. Few classes of drugs, however, have been shown to extend life significantly and there are cost savings to be made in other areas of prescribing (for example, anti-ulcer drugs and non-steroidal anti-inflammatories). Inevitably statin costs will reduce and cost effectiveness will increase.

Table 12.3 gives an indication of drug costs at current (1997) prices in the UK.

Commissioning services for the prevention and treatment of CHD

The scale of the problem and the impact of the mortality and morbidity involved make CHD prevention and treatment the major health priority in all parts of the UK. Local agreements for service provision must balance sophisticated medical interventions, such as revascularization procedures, against the health gains of other forms of prevention and care, some of which may be of less proved effectiveness. Commissioning of services should ideally be evidence based, aimed at local priorities and the Health of the Nation targets, and reflecting the increased role of primary care. Only in primary care can the major burden of continuing primary and secondary prevention be addressed.

Moreover, primary care teams are now able to influence the provision of services for their parents either directly through purchasing (either fundholding or locally based purchasing) or indirectly through advisory roles to commissioning agencies. Primary care thus finds itself at the centre of a coordinated programme for CHD prevention and treatment (Figure 12.1).

Whilst the effectiveness of some forms of health promotion in primary prevention is unproven, much of the fall in CHD death rates since the 1970s is attributable to CHD risk factor reductions. The evidence for secondary prevention is strong, particularly for cholesterol lowering, cessation of smoking, BP reduction and the use of other drugs such as aspirin, beta-blockers and ACE inhibitors in heart failure. Targeting secondary prevention first will produce short-term gains, primary prevention being a longer-term strategy. Unfortunately 75% of those with CHD under 65 are first diagnosed when they

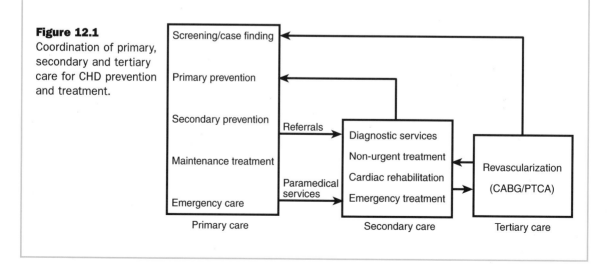

Figure 12.1
Coordination of primary, secondary and tertiary care for CHD prevention and treatment.

have a heart attack. As 25% of people with heart attacks die before reaching hospital, secondary prevention is not always applicable.

The care of the patient with myocardial infarction can be improved in terms of prioritized ambulance dispatch, improved CPR education and high technology hospital facilities. The needs of the elderly, women and certain ethnic groups (e.g. South Asians) need to be addressed. Services for angina (improved access to exercise ECG, angiography and rapid assessment clinics) and for heart failure (improved access to echocardiography) should be reviewed. There is considerable variation in the provision of cardiac rehabilitation and revascularization services. For example, few districts in the UK achieve British Cardiac Society norms for revascularization (600 CABG and 400 PTCA per year per million population).

If primary care teams can work with health authorities to produce a strategy responsive to individual needs with effective prevention programmes, major falls in CHD mortality and morbidity will result.

Case studies

The following 20 case studies represent practical examples from our experience of assessing coronary risk and the need for intervention in patients with varying risk factor profiles. The lipid profiles are measured in mmol/l (Figure 13.1) and can be assumed to represent fasting levels.

The reader should evaluate each patient's global risk by multifactorial risk assessment and formulate a management plan, which should include not only a strategy (e.g. change diet, stop smoking, add medication) but also an idea of the 'aggression' of the intervention required to reduce global risk. Plans should be realistic and achievable and should reflect the evidence base of modern clinical practice.

A commentary from the authors is provided after the case studies.

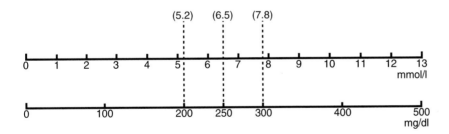

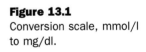

Figure 13.1
Conversion scale, mmol/l to mg/dl.

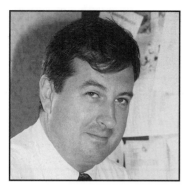

CASE 1
48-year-old director

Coronoary angioplasty 1 year ago	TC	6.3
Ex-smoker	HDL	1.1
BP 146/88	TG	1.9
No family history		
BMI 26		
Alcohol 26 units per week		
Aspirin		

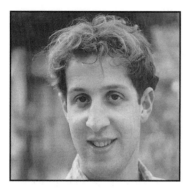

CASE 2
27-year-old actor

Non-smoker	TC	9.5
BP 124/62	HDL	1.0
Father died MI at 49 years of age	TG	1.1
Paternal granddfather died suddenly at 50 years of age		
Brother angina 40 years of age		
Wife just had twins		
Tendon xanthomata		

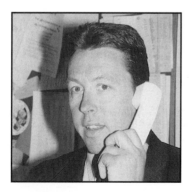

CASE 3
45-year-old banker

Smokes 15 a day	TC	7.6
BP 170/102	HDL	1.1
Maternal uncle angina	TG	2.5
BMI 28		
Alcohol 14 units a week		

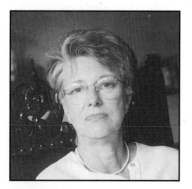

CASE 4
58-year-old headmistress

Smokes 20 a day	TC	8.2
BP 144/86	HDL	1.3
Mother angina/ccf	TG	2.1
Maternal aunt MI 65 years of age		
BMI 24		
No alcohol		

Authors' comments

CASE 1

JMM This patient has already proved his atherosclerotic potential at a relatively young age and is at high risk of a further CHD event. The ASPIRE study shows us that many patients who might benefit from secondary prevention do not receive appropriate advice. I would reinforce the lifestyle messages regarding diet and exercise that this patient should already have received but institute medication if there was no further improvement in lipid parameters after three months.

DJB Based on 4S and CARE studies, he will benefit from aggressive therapy with a statin. His calculated LDL cholesterol is currently 4.3 mmol/l and this should be reduced to below 2.6 mmol/l. Moderating his alcohol intake would help to reduce his BMI and his blood pressure. This is just the sort of patient who needs to be identified and treated and is the top priority in the British Hyperlipidaemia Association guidelines.

CASE 2

JMM Familial hypercholesterolaemia (FH) is one of the commonest inherited conditions, affecting 1 in 500 patients. Here there is a clear family history of early coronary death, there are obvious physical signs and high levels of LDL. Diet and medication are appropriate but I would consider referral to a specialist centre for advice.

DJB This patient is best managed in a specialist lipid clinic. He will probably require a combination of simvastatin (40 mg/day at bedtime) and a resin such as cholestyramine (two sachets before dinner). I would arrange non-invasive cardiac testing every two years and have a low threshold for referral for angiography. Family screening is mandatory. For research purposes I would arrange DNA testing for LDL receptor mutations and the possibility of familial defective apoprotein B. If a mutation is identified this will facilitate definitive family screening.

CASE 3

JMM Multiple risk factors are active here, including the pattern of mixed hyperlipidaemia. There is plenty of scope for lifestyle change including the management of hypertension, cessation of smoking and dietary alteration. Losing weight may improve blood pressure and lipid levels and increasing exercise might facilitate this. If progressive improvement in global risk cannot be demonstrated in 6–9 months, I would start lipid-lowering medication.

DJB In primary prevention it is important to assess individual risk before making a decision on drug therapy. His mixed dyslipidaemia together with two other major risk factors and a family history put him into a risk category where drug therapy is justified if lifestyle measures fail. I would also measure his fibrinogen and Lp(a) as further risk indicators. Based on evidence from the WOSCOPS trial I would recommend a statin.

CASE 4

JMM This lady could improve her risk profile significantly by stopping smoking. Her lipid levels are high at a time that rates of CHD for women begin to exceed those of men. I would concentrate on lifestyle change and consider the role of HRT before lipid-lowering medication.

DJB She does have a family history of CHD and she should be actively helped to give up cigarettes. Combination HRT is a first-line therapeutic option and will reduce her LDL cholesterol and also protect in other ways. Transdermal oestrogen will not exacerbate the hypertriglyceridaemia and may even decrease it.

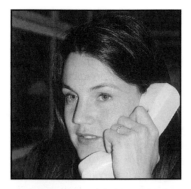

29-year-old secretary

Non-smoker	TC	11.0
BP 110/60	HDL	1.4
Father MI at 39 years of age	TG	12.6
BMI 22		
Tubero eruptive xanthomata		

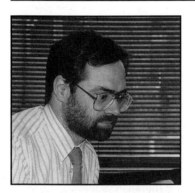

41-year-old programmer

Smokes 20 a day	Turbid	
BP 116/74	TC	9.0
No family history	HDL	0.9
BMI 26	TG	23.7
Alcohol 7 units a week		
Recurrent abdominal pain		

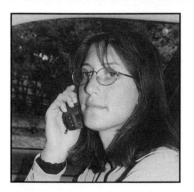

27-year-old banker

Non-smoker	TC	12.2
BP 114/80	HDL	0.9
Mother MI 52 years of age	TG	3.8
Maternal uncle MI 46 years of age		
Maternal grandfather MI 48 years of age		
Early xanthelasma		

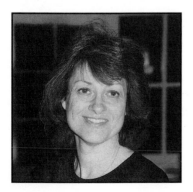

44-year-old housewife

Non-smoker	TC	7.4
BP 140/82	HDL	3.0
No family history	TG	1.6
BMI 28		

CASE 5

JMM From a family history of early coronary death, the suspicion that a genetic defect might be active is confirmed by the finding of tubero-eruptive xanthomata on this patient's elbows and the grossly abnormal lipid profile. Despite its rarity, remnant hyperlipidaemia is to be found in family practice and the metabolic and physical abnormalities respond well to treatment.

DJB Remnant hyperlipidaemia (dysbetalipoproteinaemia type III) is rare but important to recognize because of the high risk of vascular disease. She should be referred to a specialist lipid clinic. She is highly likely to demonstrate E2 homozygosity; her VLDL isolated by ultracentrifugation will show an increased cholesterol/triglyceride ratio and her lipoprotein electrophoresis a broad-beta pattern. She probably has familial combined hyperlipidaemia in addition to E2 homozygosity leading to the type III phenotype. Family screening would be worthwhile. Lifestyle measures can be quite effective in this condition but drug therapy may be required. I would suggest gemfibrozil (1.2 g/day). Her xanthomata will regress with treatment. She will need to be counselled with regard to effective contraception and the drug will need to be stopped prior to planned conception. Careful monitoring of triglyceride levels will be required during pregnancy.

CASE 6

JMM Plasma becomes milky in appearance when triglyceride content exceeds about 11 mmol/l. Triglyceride levels in excess of 10 mmol/l increase the likelihood of acute pancreatitis, which may be the explanation for this patient's abdominal pain.

DJB He has the type V phenotype with hyperchylomicronaemia and raised VLDL as indicated by the raised cholesterol. He should be referred to a specialist centre. Severe hypertriglyceridaemia is most commonly due to secondary causes, particularly alcohol and diabetes. He does not drink to excess but it is important to check his glucose. Occasionally this phenotype can run in families and is described as familial hypertriglyceridaemia. It is likely that lipoprotein lipase or apoprotein C2 deficiency would have presented at an earlier age. This can be confirmed by the rapid response to a very low fat diet and the measurement of lipoprotein lipase enzyme activity. Familial hypertriglyceridaemia does not respond rapidly to diet and lipoprotein lipase activity is measurable.

Treatment is with a low fat, low refined carbohydrate diet together with fish oil (MaxEpa, 10 capsules/day) plus a fibrate.

CASE 7

JMM The revelation of an adverse family history in a patient with a severe mixed hyperlipidaemia suggests the possibility of familial combined hyperlipidaemia. More common than FH, presentation is in adult life and differentiation from 'common' hyperlipidaemia is sometimes difficult.

DJB She should be referred to the lipid clinic. Given the family history and this lipid phenotype she could have FH or FCH. Tendon xanthomata on her or a family member would point to FH, as these do not occur in FCH. Genetic studies of the LDL receptor might help if a receptor mutation is found. Screening the surviving family might show the differing lipoprotein phenotypes typical of FCH. Unfortunately there is as yet no definitive marker of this condition.

Treatment is the same. She needs high-dose statin together with diet and lifestyle measures. Non-invasive cardiac monitoring is also important. Occasionally combined therapy of statin plus fibrate is required.

CASE 8

JMM Occasionally families are encountered where levels of HDL are very high. High HDL is associated with longevity and although the total cholesterol is raised the patient can be safely reassured.

DJB She has a substantial HDL cholesterol and a calculated LDL of 3.7 mmol/l. This patient demonstrates the importance of performing a full lipid profile.

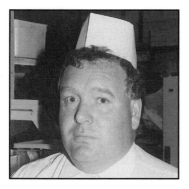

CASE 9
38-year-old chef

Non-smoker	TC	9.4
BP 160/90	HDL	1.6
No family history	TG	3.8
BMI 34		
Alcohol 15 units a week		
Xanthelasmata		

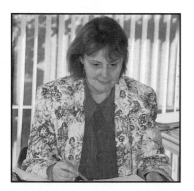

CASE 10
40-year-old businesswoman

Smokes 5 a day	TC	8.4
BP 130/82	HDL	1.4
Maternal grandfather CVA	TG	2.6
BMI 28 (was 23)		
Alcohol 10 units a week		

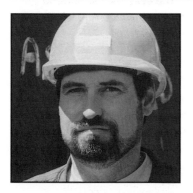

CASE 11
49-year-old labourer

Smokes 10 a day	TC	7.8
BP 170/100	HDL	1.7
No family history	TG	4.4
BMI 29		
Alcohol 56 units a week		
Xanthelasmata		

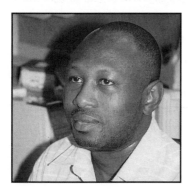

CASE 12
43-year-old transport manager

Non-smoker	TC	7.6
Hypertensive on thiazide and betablocker	HDL	0.9
No family history	TG	2.9

CASE 9

JMM This patient's mixed hyperlipidaemia almost certainly relates to his obesity. Xanthelasmata, whilst very non-specific, often correlate with elevated triglyceride levels, which in turn are often markers of obesity or excessive alcohol consumption. I would concentrate on weight reduction by realistic goal setting and supportive follow-up.

DJB He is markedly obese with mixed hyperlipidaemia but a reasonable HDL – perhaps he is drinking more than he admits to. It is important to check his glucose and thyroid function. Weight reduction is the first line of therapy.

CASE 10

JMM Hypothyroidism is common and often difficult to diagnose without an index of suspicion. This patient's TSH was elevated and lipid levels made a prompt reduction when treatment with thyroxine was started.

DJB In my lipid clinic I discover unsuspected hypothyroidism in about six patients a year. Although typically associated with hypercholesterolaemia, it can cause any lipid abnormality.

CASE 11

JMM This is the typical mixed hyperlipidaemia often associated with alcohol abuse. Whilst potentially 'cardioprotective' at lower amounts, higher alcohol consumption is associated with increased CHD. Lifestyle change might improve this patient's BP and BMI as well as his lipid profile.

DJB High alcohol intake increases both triglyceride and HDL – usually these parameters are inversely related. He needs to reduce his alcohol intake substantially.

CASE 12

JMM The blood pressure of Afro-Caribbeans is notoriously difficult to control with beta-blockers and ACE inhibitors. As both thiazides (in standard dose) and beta-blockers have adverse effects on lipid metabolism, I would use an alpha-blocker or a long-acting calcium antagonist. Formulations of very low dose thiazides are still awaited.

DJB His HDL is below the tenth centile and the combination of hypertriglyceridaemia and an LDL/HDL of greater than 5 puts him at high risk – he has the so-called atherogenic profile. The beta-blocker (if it does not have vasodilator properties) is likely to exacerbate his hypertriglyceridaemia and low HDL. The thiazide at high dose (5 mg or greater) will exacerbate the hypercholesterolaemia and the hypertriglyceridaemia. It is important to exclude glucose intolerance. I still use thiazides but at doses of 2.5 mg/day or less. The alpha-blocker is a good idea.

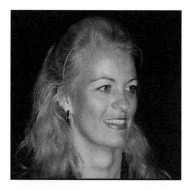

CASE 13
37-year-old dress designer

Non-smoker	TC	6.2
BP 130/80	HDL	0.9
No family history	TG	2.5
BMI 22		
Diabetes mellitus on insulin		

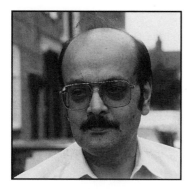

CASE 14
38-year-old garage worker

Indian	TC	7.3
Non-smoker	HDL	0.7
BP 170/100 NIDDM	TG	3.8
Paternal uncles × 2 MI		
BMI 25 WHR 1.3		
Xanthelasmata and arcus		

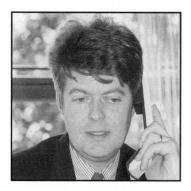

CASE 15
42-year-old doctor

Non-smoker	TC	7.8
Hypertensive on ACE inhibitor	HDL	1.4
Father PVD	TG	3.1
BMI 27		
Alcohol 36 units a week		

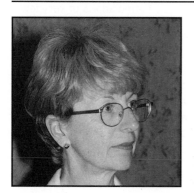

CASE 16
48-year-old teacher

Smokes 25 a day	TC	7.6
BP 90/50	HDL	1.0
No family history	TG	1.7
No alcohol		
Amenorrhoea		

CASE 13

JMM For a woman, diabetes removes any sex-related benefit in CHD prevention. Here we see the common pattern amongst diabetics of low HDL with elevated triglyceride. After attention to lifestyle, despite the only moderately raised cholesterol level, I would consider medication.

DJB I would want to assess her diabetic control carefully as it is unusual for an IDDM patient to have such a low HDL. Usually HDL is normal or even increased in IDDM. Similarly the raised triglyceride suggests poor control. It would be important to check for proteinuria as lipid abnormalities tend to develop with nephropathy. She should be referred to the diabetic clinic.

CASE 14

JMM The clustering of hypertension, diabetes, central obesity, low HDL and elevated triglycerides suggests the presence of the insulin resistance syndrome. Besides the specific management of diabetes and hypertension, attention to diet and encouraging weight loss and exercise are important.

DJB This man is at high risk of premature vascular disease. He needs aggressive therapy. Anti-hypertensive and hypolipidaemic agents may be required if attention to glycaemic control and lifestyle measures fail. I would treat his NIDDM with metformin and acarbose and the lipids (if necessary) with a fibrate. I would use an ACE inhibitor for his blood pressure.

CASE 15

JMM Again we see a pattern of mixed hyperlipidaemia in an individual with some lifestyle change to make. Having cut alcohol consumption and lost weight, decisions must be made regarding lipid-lowering therapy if the profile remains unaltered.

DJB I would want to know at what age his father developed vascular disease and whether he had any known major risk factors – particularly, was he a smoker or diabetic? The most important initial management is reduction in alcohol intake and reduction in weight. It is important to check his glucose.

CASE 16

JMM It is likely that this lady is perimenopausal. Having excluded a secondary cause such as hypothyroidism, she still has an elevated total cholesterol level. Her HDL level is low and TC : HDL ratio is 7.6. Clearly she should stop smoking but I would be keen to discuss with her the benefits of HRT.

DJB It is unusual to see such a low HDL in a woman. I would agree with the suggestion of HRT and would use transdermal oestrogen. It would be interesting to see the effect of smoking cessation on her HDL – it should rise.

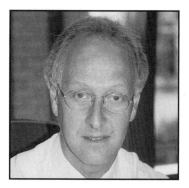

CASE 17
55-year-old store manager

Ex-smoker 1 year	TC	7.7
BP 124/80	HDL	1.1
Brother angina 62 years of age	TG	2.0
Asymptomatic aortic aneurysm		
Arcus senilis		

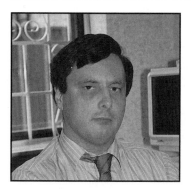

CASE 18
48-year-old company secretary

Ex-smoker 3 years (since first MI)	TC	5.2
BP 134/68	HDL	0.7
Father has angina 73 years of age	TG	1.3

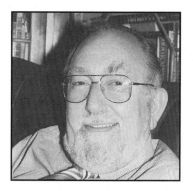

CASE 19
63-year-old teacher

Ex-smoker 1 month (since MI 1	TC	4.9
month ago)	HDL	1.4
BP 160/92	TG	1.4
No family history		
BMI 28		

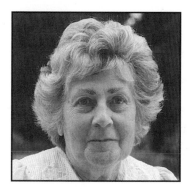

CASE 20
72-year-old retired

Non-smoker	TC	8.8
BP 155/74	HDL	1.4
Brother died MI 58 years old	TG	1.8
NIDDM		

CASE 17

JMM The role of cholesterol lowering in peripheral vascular disease is much less established than in CHD. This man, however, is more likely to die of CHD than his peripheral atherosclerosis and merits intervention. Life style measures and drug treatment are likely to be necessary.

DJB This man would fit the West of Scotland primary prevention study and is likely to benefit from lipid-lowering drug therapy. I would prescribe a statin if life style measures fail.

CASE 18

JMM Here is another case of secondary prevention in a man who had an MI at a relatively young age. The apparently low total cholesterol disguises the low HDL level and the unsatisfactorily high calculated LDL value of 3.9. I would use a fibrate in addition to the usual lifestyle advice.

DJB I think I would disagree on the choice of a fibrate. In my experience cases of isolated low HDL cholesterol do not respond to a fibrate. I would use a statin to reduce his LDL to 2 mmol/l.

CASE 19

JMM It seems surprising that this man should have suffered a heart attack with his apparently innocuous risk factor profile. Lipid levels taken following major illness, however, do not always reflect pre-event status and measurements should be repeated in two months time.

DJB He certainly needs further assessment in a couple of months and I would wager that his cholesterol will rise and he will need a statin.

CASE 20

JMM Although the relative benefits of cholesterol lowering in the elderly may be reduced, the absolute benefits may be greater (because the elderly have more CHD events). Few studies have included trial subjects over 70 years old. In this elderly lady I would not proceed beyond lifestyle advice.

DJB I certainly treat elderly people with established CHD as the benefits are seen relatively early. For primary prevention it is a matter of judgement. More clinical trials are needed in this area.

References

Abbott, R.D., Donahue, R.P., Kannel, W.B. and Wilson, P.W. (1988) The impact of diabetes on survival following myocardial infarction in men vs women. The Framingham Study. *J. Am. Med. Assoc.* **260**, 3456–3460.

Alberti, K.G.M.M. and Gries, F.A. (1988) Management of NIDDM. Report of the European Working Group. *Diabetic Med.* **5**, 275–281.

Altschul, R., Hoffer, A. and Stephen, J.D. (1955) Influence of nicotinic acid on serum cholesterol in man. *Arch. Biochem. Biophys.* **54**, 558–9.

Amery, A. *et al.* (1985) Mortality and morbidity results from the European Working Party on High Blood Pressure in the Elderly Trial. *Lancet.* **i**, 1349–54.

Anderson, T.J., Meredith I.T., Yeung, A.C. *et al.* (1995) The effect of cholesterol lowering and antioxidant therapy on endothelium-dependent coronary vasomotion. *N. Engl. J. Med.* **332**, 488–493.

Andrews, T.C., Raby, K., Barry, J. *et al.* (1997) Effect of cholesterol reduction on myocardial ischaemia in patients with coronary disease. *Circulation.* **95**, 324–8.

ASPIRE Steering Group (1996) A British Cardiac Society survey of the potential for the secondary prevention of coronary disease – ASPIRE (Action on Secondary Prevention through Intervention to Reduce Events). *Heart* **75**, 334.

Assman, G. *et al.* (1991) The Prospective Cardiovascular Münster Study. *Am. J. Cardiol.* **68**, 30A–34A.

Austin, M.A., Breslow, J.L., Hennekens, C.H. *et al.* (1988) Low density lipoprotein subclass patterns and risk of myocardial infarction. *J. Am. Med. Assoc.* **260**, 1917–21.

Barbir, M. Khaghani, A., Kehely, A. *et al.* (1992) Normal levels of lipoproteins including lipoprotein(a) after liver–heart transplantation in a patient with homozygous familial hypercholesterolaemia. *Quart. J. Med.* **85**, 807–812.

Barrett-Connor, E. and Wingard, D.L. (1983) Sex differential in ischaemic heart disease mortality in diabetics: a prospective population-based study. *Am. J. Epidemiol.* **118**, 489–496.

Barth, J.D., Arntzemus, A.C. and Kromhout, D. (1987) Follow up on the Leiden Trial. *N. Engl. J. Med.* **316**, 881–882.

Beaumont, J.L., Carlson, L.A., Cooper, G.R. *et al.* (1970) Classification of hyperlipidaemia and hyperlipoproteinaemias. *Bull. WHO* **43**, 891–915.

Ball, M. and Mann, J. (1994) *Lipids and Heart Disease: a Guide for the Primary Care Team*, Oxford Medical Press, Oxford.

Betteridge, D.J., Dodson, P.M., Durrington, P. *et al.* (1993) Management of hyperlipidaemia: guidelines of the British Hyperlipidaemia Association. *Postgrad Med. J.* **69**, 359–369.

Black, D. (1994) Atorvastatin: a step ahead for HMG-CoA reductase inhibitors. *Atherosclerosis.* **109**, 88–9.

Blankenhorn, D.H., Nession, S.A., Johnson, R.L. *et al.* (1987) Beneficial effects of combined colestipol–niacin therapy on coronary atherosclerosis and coronary venous bypass grafts. *J. Am. Med. Assoc.* **257**, 3233–3240.

Blankenhorn, D.H., Azen, S.P., Karmsch, D.M. *et al.* (1993) Coronary angiographic changes with lovastatin therapy. The Monitored Atherosclerosis Regression Study (MARS). *Ann. Intern. Med.* **119**, 969–976.

Boaz, A., Kaduskar, S. and Rayner, M. (1996) *Coronary Heart Disease Statistics*, British Heart Foundation Statistics Database, London.

Borsch-Johnsen, K. and Kreiner, S. (1987) Proteinuria: value as a predictor of cardiovascular mortality in insulin dependent diabetes mellitus *Br. Med. J.* **294**, 1651–1654.

Brensike, J.F., Levy, R.I., Kelsey, S.F. *et al.* (1984) Effects of cholestyramine on progression of coronary atherosclerosis: results of the NHLBI Type II Coronary Intervention Study. *Circulation* **69**, 313–324.

Brown, G., Albers, J.J., Fisher, L.D. *et al.* (1990) Regression of coronary artery disease as a result of intensive lipid lowering therapy in men with high levels of apolipoprotein B. *N. Engl. J. Med.* **323**, 1289–1298.

Brown, G., Zhao, Z.-Q., Sacco, D.J. *et al.* (1993) Lipid lowering and plaque regression: new insights into prevention of plaque disruption and clinical events in coronary disease. *Circulation* **87**, 1781–1791.

Brown, M.S. and Goldstein, J.L. (1983) Lipoprotein metabolism in the macrophage. *Ann. Rev. Biochem.* **52**, 223–61.

Brown, M.S. and Goldstein, J.L. (1986) Receptor-mediated control of cholesterol metabolism. *Science* **191**, 150–154.

Buchwald, H. (1964) Lowering cholesterol absorption and blood levels by ileal exclusion. *Circulation* **29**, 713–720.

Buchwald, H., Varco, R.L., Matts, J.P. *et al.* (1990) Effect of partial ileal bypass surgery on mortality and morbidity from coronary heart disease in patients with hypercholesterolaemia: report of the Programme on the Surgical Control of the Hyperlipidaemias (POSCH). *N. Engl. J. Med.* **323**, 946–955.

Burr, M.L. *et al* (1989) Effects of change in fat, fish and fibre intakes on death and myocardial infarction: Death and Reinfarction Trial (DART). *Lancet.* **ii**, 757–60.

Carlson, L.A. and Rosenhamer, G. (1988) Reduction of mortality in the Stockholm Ischaemic Heart Disease Secondary Prevention Study by combined treatment with clofibrate and nicotinic acid. *Acta Med. Scand.* **223**, 405–418.

Cashin-Hemphill, L., Mack, W.J., Pogoda, J.M. *et al.* (1990) Beneficial effects of colestipol niacin on coronary atherosclerosis. A 4-year follow up. *J. Am. Med. Assoc.* **264**, 3013–3017.

Collins, R., Peto, R., MacMahon, S. *et al.* (1990) Blood pressure, stroke, and coronary heart disease. Part 2. Short-term reductions in blood pressure: overview of randomised drug trials in the epidemiological context. *Lancet* **335**, 827–838.

Committee of Principal Investigators (1978) Report on a cooperative trial in the primary prevention of ischaemic heart disease using clofibrate. *Br. Heart J.* **40**, 1069–1118.

Consensus Statement (1993) Detection and management of lipid disorders in diabetes. *Diabetes Care* **16**, 106–112.

Coope, J. and Warrender, T.S. (1986) Randomized trial of treatment of hypertension in elderly patients in primary care. *Br. Med. J.* **293**, 1143–8.

Coronary Drug Project Research Group (1975) The Coronary Drug Project: clofibrate and niacin in coronary heart disease. *J. Am. Med. Assoc.* **231**, 360–381.

Crouse, J.R., Byington, R.P., Bond, M.G. *et al.* (1995) Pravastatin lipids and atherosclerosis in the carotid arteries (PLAC-II). *Am. J. Cardiol.* **75**, 455–459.

Dahlof, B. *et al.* (1991) Morbidity and mortality in the Swedish Trial in Old Patients with Hypertension (STOP – Hypertension). *Lancet.* **338**, 1281–5.

Davidson, M.H., Stein, E.A., Dujovne, C.A. *et al.* (1997). The efficacy and six-week tolerability of simvastatin 80 mg and 160 mg/day. *Am. J. Cardiol.* **79**, 38–42.

Davies, M.J. (1996) Stability and instability: two faces of coronary atherosclerosis. The Paul Dudley White Lecture 1995. *Circulation.* **94**, 2013–20.

Davies, M.J. and Thomas, T. (1981) The pathological basis and micro-anatomy of occlusive thrombosis formation in human coronary arteries. Philosophical Transactions of the Royal Society of London, Series B. *Biological Sciences (London).* **294**, 225–9.

Davignon, J., Gregg, R.E. and Sing, C.F. (1988) Apolipoprotein E polymorphism and atherosclerosis. *Arteriosclerosis* **8**, 1–21.

Dayton, S., Pearce, M.L., Hashimoto, S. *et al.* (1969) A controlled clinical trial of a diet high in unsaturated fat in preventing complications of atherosclerosis. *Circulation* **XXXIX** (Suppl. II), II-1–II-60.

Deegan, P. and Feely, J. (1996) Making sensible drug choices – horses for courses, in *Lipids: Current Perspectives* (ed. D.J. Betteridge), Martin Dunitz, London.

Diabetes Control and Complications Trial Research Group (1993) Effect of intensive treatment of diabetes on the development and progression of longterm complications in insulin dependent diabetes mellitus. *N. Engl. J. Med.* **329**, 977–986.

Doll, R. and Peto, R. (1976) Mortality in relation to smoking: 20 years observation of British doctors. *Br. Med. J.* 4, 1525.

Duffield, R.G.M., Lewis, B., Miller, N.E. *et al.* (1983) Treatment of hyperlipidaemia retards progression of symptomatic femoral athero-sclerosis. *Lancet* ii, 639–643.

Durrington, P.M. (1995) *Hyperlipidaemia: Diagnosis and Management*, 2nd edn, Butterworth Heinemann, Oxford.

Ericsson, C.G., Hamsten, A., Nilsson, J. *et al.* (1996) Angiographic assessment of effects of bezafibrate on progression of coronary artery disease in young male postinfarction patients. *Lancet* **347**, 849–853.

European Atherosclerosis Society (1992) Prevention of coronary heart disease: scientific background and new clinical guidelines. Recommenda-tions of the European Atherosclerosis Society prepared by the Inter-national Task Force for Prevention of Coronary Heart Disease. *Nutr. Metab. Cardiovasc. Dis.* **2**, 113–156.

Farmer, J.A. and Gotto, A.M. (1995) Currently available hypolipidaemic drugs and future therapeutic developments, in *Baillière's Clinical Endocri-nology and Metabolism*, Vol. 9, No. 4, *Dyslipidaemia* (ed. D.J. Betteridge), Baillière Tindall, London.

Frick, M.H., Elo, O., Haapa, K. *et al.* (1987) The Helsinki Heart Study: primary prevention trial with gemofibrozil in middle-aged men with dyslipidaemia. Safety of treatment, changes in risk factors and incidence of coronary heart disease. *N. Engl. J. Med.* **317**, 1237–1245.

Friedewald, W.T., Levy, R. and Frederickson, D.S. (1972) Estimation of the concentration of low density lipoprotein cholesterol in plasma without use of the preparative ultracentrifuge. *Clin. Chem.* **18**, 499–502.

Furberg, C.D., Adams, H.P., Applegate, W.B. *et al.*, for the Asymptomatic Carotid Artery Progression Study (ACAPS) Research Group (1994) Effect of lovastatin on early carotid atherosclerosis and cardiovascular events. *Circulation* **90**, 1679–1687.

Furberg, B. and Furberg, C. (1994) What clinicians need to know about clinical trials. In *All That Glitters is Not Gold*. Dr Potata, Winston-Salem, USA.

Garrow, J.S. (1981) *Treat Obesity Seriously*, Churchill Livingstone.

Goldstein, J.L., Hazzard, W.R., Schrott, H.G. *et al.* (1973) Hyperlipidaemia in coronary heart disease II. Genetic analysis of lipid levels in 176 families and delineation of a new inherited disorder: combined hyperlipidaemia. *J. Clin. Invest.* **54**, 1544–1568.

Grossman, M., Raper, S.E., Kozarsky, K. *et al.* (1994 Successful ex vivo gene therapy directed to liver in a patient with familial hypercholesterolaemia. *Nature Genet.* **6**, 335–341.

Hambrecht, R., Niebauer, J., Marburger, C. *et al.* (1993) Various intensities of leisure time physical activity in patients with coronary artery disease: effects on cardiorespiratory fitness and progression of coronary atherosclerotic lesions. *J. Am. Coll. Cardiol.* **22**, 468–477.

Havel, R.J. and Kane, J.P. (1995) Structure and metabolism of plasma hypoproteins, in *The Metabolic and Molecular Bases of Inherited Disease* (eds. C.R. Scriver *et al.*), 7th edn, McGraw Hill, New York.

Heady, J.A., Morris, J.N. and Oliver, M.F. (1992) WHO clofibrate/cholesterol trial: clarifications. *Lancet* **340**, 1405–1406.

Hehmann, H.W., Bunt, T., Hellwig, N. *et al.* (1991) Progression and regression of minor coronary arterial narrowings by quantitative angiography after fenofibrate therapy. *Am. J. Cardiol.* **67**, 957–961.

Hjermann, I., Holme, I., Velve Byre K. and Leren, P. (1981) Effect of diet and smoking intervention on the incidence of coronary heart disease: report from the Oslo Study Group of a randomised trial in healthy men. *Lancet* **ii**, 1303–1310.

Holme, I. (1990) An analysis of randomized trials evaluating the effect of cholesterol reduction in total mortality and coronary heart disease incidence. *Circulation* **82**, 1916–1924.

Humphries, S.E., Dunning, A., Xu C.-F. *et al.* (1992) DNA polymorphism studies: approaches to elucidating multifactorial ischaemic heart disease: the apoB gene as an example. *Ann. Med.* **24**, 349–356.

Illingworth, D.R. and Tobert, J.A. (1994) A review of clinical trials comparing HMG-CoA reductase inhibitors. *Clin. Thera.* **16**, 366–85.

Innerarity, J.L., Mahley, R.W., Weisgraber, K.H. *et al.* (1990) Familial defective apolipoprotein B-100: a mutation of apolipoprotein B that causes hypercholesterolaemia. *J. Lipid Res.* **31**, 1337–1349.

International Task Force for Prevention of Coronary Heart Disease (1992) Prevention of coronary heart disease: scientific background and new clinical guidelines. Recommendations of the European Atherosclerosis Society. *Nutr. Metab. Cardiovasc. Dis.* **2**, 113–156.

Jackson, R. *et al.* (1991) Alcohol consumption and risk of coronary heart disease. *Br. Med. J.* **303**, 211–16.

Johannesson, M., Jonsson, B., Kjekshus, J. *et al.* (1997) Cost effectiveness of simvastatin treatment to lower cholesterol levels in patients with coronary heart disease. *N. Engl. J. Med.* **336**, 332–6.

Jonsson, B., Johannesson, M., Kjekshus, J. *et al.* (1996) Cost effectiveness of cholesterol lowering. *Eur. Heart J.* **17**, 1001–7.

Kane, J.P., Malloy, M.J., Ports, T.H.A. *et al.* (1990) Regression of coronary atherosclerosis during treatment of familial hypercholesterolaemia with combined drug regimens. *J. Am. Med. Assoc.* **264**, 3007–3012.

Kannel, W.B. (1983) High density lipoproteins: epidemiologic profile and risks of coronary artery disease. *Am. J. Cardiol.* **52**, 9B–12B.

Kannell, W.B. and McGee, D.I. (1979) Diabetes and glucose tolerance as risk factors for cardiovascular disease. The Framingham Study. *Diabetes Care* **2**, 120–126.

Keys, A. (1980) *Seven Countries: a multivariate analysis of death and coronary heart disease*, Harvard University Press.

Koskinen, P., Manttari, M., Manninen, V. *et al.* (1992) Coronary heart disease incidence in NIDDM patients in the Helsinki Heart Study. *Diabetes Care* **15**, 820–825.

Kraus, H.M.J. *et al.* (eds) (1992) *The St Vincent Declaration. Diabetes Care and Research in Europe*, WHO, Geneva.

Krauss, R.M. and Burke, D.J. (1982) Identification of multiple subclasses of plasma low density lipoproteins in normal humans. *J. Lipid Res.* **23**, 97–104.

Krone, W. and Müller-Wieland, D. (1990) Hyperlipidaemia and hypertension, in *Baillière's Clinical Endocrinology and Metabolism*, Vol. 4, No. 4 (ed. D.J. Betteridge), Baillière Tindall, London.

Krowlewski, A.S., Kosinski, E.J., Warram, J.H. *et al.* (1989) Magnitude and determinants of coronary artery disease in juvenile onset insulin dependent diabetes mellitus. *Am. J. Cardiol.* **59**, 750–755.

Krumholz, H.M., Seeman, T.E., Merrill, S.S. *et al.* (1994) Lack of association between cholesterol and coronary heart disease mortality and morbidity and all cause mortality in persons older than 70 years. *J. Am. Med. Assoc.* **272**, 1335–1340.

Law, M.R., Wald, N.J., Wu, T. *et al.* (1994a) The Cholesterol Papers I–III. *Br. Med. J.* **308**, 363–379.

Law, M.R., Wald, N.J. and Thompson, S.G. (1994b) By how much and how quickly does reduction in serum cholesterol concentration lower risk of ischaemic heart disease? *Br. Med. J.* **308**, 367–372.

Law, M.R., Thompson, S.G. and Wald, N.J. (1994c) Assessing possible hazards of reducing serum cholesterol. *Br. Med. J.* **308**, 373–379.

Leung, W.-H., Lau, C.-P. and Wong, C.-K. (1993) Beneficial effect of cholesterol-lowering therapy on coronary endothelium-dependent relaxation in hypercholesterolaemic patients. *Lancet* **341**, 1496–1500.

Lipid Research Clinics Programme (1984) The Lipid Research Clinics Coronary Primary Prevention Trial Results I. Reduction in incidence of coronary heart disease. *J. Am. Med. Assoc.* **251**, 351–364.

MacMahon, S.W., Macdonald, G.J. and Blacket, R.B. (1985) Plasma lipoprotein levels in treated and untreated hypertensive men and women. The National Heart Foundation of Australia risk factor prevalence study. *Aerterioscler. Thromb.* **5**, 391–396.

Margolis, J.R., Kennal, W.B., Feinleib, M. *et al.* Clinical features of unrecognized myocardial infarction; silent and symptomatic. Eighteen year follow up. The Framingham Study. *Am. J. Cardiol.* **32**, 1–7.

Marmot, M.G. *et al.* (1991) Health inequalities among British civil servants: the Whitehall II study. *Lancet.* **338**, 1387–93.

MASS Investigators (1994) Effect of simvastatin on coronary atheroma: The Multicentre Anti Atheroma Study (MAAS). *Lancet* **344**, 633–638.

McKeigue, P.M. *et al.* (1991) Relation of central obesity and insulin resistance with high diabetes prevalence and cardiovascular risk in South Asians. *Lancet.* **337**, 382–6.

Meade, T.W. *et al.* (1986) Haemostatic function and ischaemic heart disease: principal results of the Northwick Part Heart Study. *Lancet,* **ii**, 533–7.

MRC Working Party (1992) Medical Research Council trial of treatment of hypertension in older adults: principal results. *Br. Med. J.* **304**, 405–12.

Muir, J. (1995) Effectiveness of health checks conducted by nurses in primary care: final results of the OXCHECK study. *Br. Med. J.* **310**, 1099–104.

Muldoon, M.F., Manuck, S.B. and Mathews, K.A. (1990) Lowering cholesterol concentrations and mortality: a quantitative review of primary prevention trials. *Br. Med. J.* **301**, 309–314.

National Cholesterol Education Program (1992) Report of the Expert Panel on Blood Cholesterol Levels in Children and Adolescents. *Paediatrics* **89**, 525–584.

National Cholesterol Education Program (1993) Detection, evaluation and treatment of high blood cholesterol in adults (Adult Treatment Panel II). National Institutes of Health, NIH Publication No. 93–3095. *Circulation* **89**, 1329–1445.

Nawrocki, J.W., Weiss, S.R., Davidson, M.H. *et al.* (1995) Reduction of LDL cholesterol by 25% to 60% in patients with primary hypercholesterolaemia by atorvastatin, a new HMG-CoA reductase inhibitor. *Arteriosclerosis and Thrombosis.* **15**, 678–82.

Neil, A., Rees, A. and Taylor, C. (eds) (1996) *Hyperlipidaemia in Childhood*, Royal College of Physicians, London.

Neil, H. *et al.* (1996) Garlic in the treatment of modern hyperlipidaemia: a controlled trial and a meta-analysis. *J.R. Coll. Phys.* **30**, 329–34.

O'Connor, P., Feely, J. and Shepherd, J. (1991) Lipid-lowering drugs. *Br. Med. J.* **300**, 667–672.

Ornish, D., Brown, S., Scherwitz, L.W. *et al.* (1990) Can lifestyle changes reverse coronary heart disease? The Lifestyle Heart Trial. *Lancet* **336**, 129–133.

Pedersen, T.R., Berg, K., Cook, T.J. *et al.* (1996) Safety and tolerability of cholesterol lowering with simvastatin during 5 years in the Scandinavian Simvastatin Survival Study. *Arch. Int. Med.* **156**, 2085–92.

Pedersen, T.R., Kjekshus, J., Berg, K. *et al.* (1996) Cholesterol lowering and the use of Healthcare Resources. Results of the Scandinavian Simvastatin Survival Study. *Circulation* **93**, 1796–1802.

Pekkanen, J., Linn, S., Heiss, G. *et al.* (1990) Ten year mortality from cardiovascular disease in relation to cholesterol level among men with and without pre-existing cardiovascular disease. *N. Engl. J. Med.* **322**, 1700–1707.

Pitt, B., Mancini, G.B.J., Ellis, S.B. *et al.* (1995) Pravastatin Limitation of Atherosclerosis in the Coronary Arteries (PLAC 1): Reduction in atherosclerosis progression and clinical events. *J. Am. Coll. Cardiol.* **26**, 1133–1139.

Post Coronary Artery Bypass Graft Trial Investigators (1997) The effect of aggressive lowering of low density lipoprotein cholesterol levels and low dose anticoagulation on obstructive changes in saphenous vein coronary artery bypass grafts. *N. Engl. J. Med.* **336**, 153–162.

Pyörälä, K., DeBacker, G., Graham, I. *et al.* (1994) Prevention of coronary heard disease in clinical practice. Recommendations of the Task Force of the European Society of Cardiology, European Atherosclerosis Society and European Society of Hypertension. *European Heart Journal* **15**, 1300–1331.

Pyörälä, K., Pedersen, T.R. and Kjekshsu, J. (1995) The effect of cholesterol lowering with simvastatin on coronary events in diabetic patients with coronary heart disease. *Diabetes* **44** (Suppl. 1), 125 (abstract).

Ramsey, L. *et al.* (1991) Dietary reduction of serum concentration: time to think again. *Br. Med. J.* **303**, 953–7.

Ravnskov, U. (1992) Cholesterol lowering trials in coronary heart disease: frequency of citation and outcome. *Br. Med. J.* **305**, 15–19.

Reckless, J. (1996) The 4S study and its pharmacoeconomic implications. *Pharmacoeconomics.* **9**(2), 101–5.

Richter, W.O., Jacob, B.G., Ritter, M.M. *et al.* (1993) Three year treatment of familial heterozygous hypercholesterolaemia by extracorporeal low density lipoprotein immunoadsorption with polyclonal apolipoprotein B antibodies. *Metabolism* **42**, 888–894.

Rifkind, B.M. (ed.) (1991) *Drug Treatment of Hyperlipidaemia*, Marcel Dekker Inc., New York.

Rimm, E. *et al.* (1996) Review of moderate alcohol consumption and reduced risk of coronary heart disease: is the effect due to beer, wine or spirits? *Br. Med. J.* **312**, 731–6.

Rossouw, J.E., Lewis, B. and Rifkind, B.M. (1990) The value of lowering cholesterol after myocardial infarction. *N. Engl. J. Med.* **323**, 1112–1119.

Sacks, F.M., Pfeffer, M.A., Moye, L.A. *et al.* (1996) The effects of pravastatin on coronary events after myocardial infarction in patients with average cholesterol levels. *N. Engl. J. Med.* **335**, 1001–1009.

Salonen, R., Nyyssonen, K., Porkkala-Sarataho, E. *et al.* (1995) A population based primary prevention trial of the effect of LDL lowering on atherosclerotic progression in carotid and femoral arteries. *Circulation* **92**, 1758–1764.

Scandinavian Simvastatin Survival Study Group (1994) Randomised trial of cholesterol-lowering in 4444 patients with coronary heart disease: the Scandinavian simvastatin survival study (4S). *Lancet* **344**, 1383–1389.

Scandinavian Simvastatin Survival Study Group (1995) Baseline serum cholesterol and treatment effect in the Scandinavian Simvastatin Survival Study (4S). *Lancet.* **345**, 1274–5.

Schulte, K–L. and Beil, S. (1996) Efficacy and tolerability of fluvastatin and simvastatin in hypercholesterolaemic patients. *Clin. Drug Invest.* **12**, 119–26.

Scientific Steering Committee, on behalf of the Simon Broome Register Group (1991) Risk of fatal coronary heart disease in familial hypercholesterolaemia. *Br. Med. J.* **303**, 893–896.

Shaper, A.G. *et al.* (1986) Identifying men at high risk of heart attacks: a strategy for use in general practice. *Br. Med. J.* **293**, 474–9.

SHEP Cooperative Research Group (1991) Prevention of stroke by antihypertensive drug treatment in older persons with isolated systolic hypertension. Final results of the systolic hypertension in the elderly person (SHEP). *J. Am. Med. Assoc.* **265**, 3255–64.

Shepherd, H.J. (1995) Fibrates and statins in the treatment of hyperlipidaemia: an appraisal of their efficacy and safety. *Eur. Heart J.* **16**, 5–13.

Shepherd, J., Cobbe, S.M., Ford, I. *et al.* (1995) Prevention of coronary heart disease with pravastatin in men with hypercholesterolaemia. *N. Engl. J. Med.* 333, 1301–1307.

Sivers, F. (1996) *Evidence Based Strategies for Secondary Prevention of Coronary Heart Disease*, Science Press.

Smith, G.D. and Pekkanen, J. (1992) Should there be a moratorium on the use of cholesterol lowering drugs? *Br. Med. J.* 304, 431–434.

Stamler, J., Vaccaro, O., Neaton, J.D. *et al.* (1993) Diabetes, other risk factors and 12 year cardiovascular mortality for men screened in the Multiple Risk Factor Intervention Trial. *Diabetes Care* 16, 434–444.

Starzl, T.E., Chase, H.P., Ahrens, E.H. *et al.* (1983) Portacaval shunt in patients with familial hypercholesterolaemia. *Ann. Surg.* 198, 273–283.

Starzl, T.E., Bilheimer, D.W., Bahnson, H.T. *et al.* (1984) Heart–liver transplantation in a patient with familial hypercholesterolaemia. *Lancet* i, 1382–1383.

Steinberg, D., Parthasarathy, S., Carew, T.E. *et al.* (1989) Beyond cholesterol: modifications of low density lipoprotein that increase its atherogenicity. *N. Engl. J. Med.* 320, 915–24.

Stephens, N. *et al.* (1996) Randomized controlled trial of Vitamin E in patients with coronary disease: Cambridge Heart Antioxidant Study (CHAOS). *Lancet.* 347, 781–6.

Thiery, Y. and Seidel, D. (1993) LDL apheresis: clinical experience and indications in the treatment of severe hypercholesterolaemia. *Transfus. Sci.* 14, 249–259.

Thompson, G.R. (1994) *A Handbook of Hyperlipidaemia*, 2nd edn, Current Science, London.

Thompson, G.R., Lowenthal, R. and Myant, N.B. (1975) Plasma exchange in the management of homozygous familial hypercholesterolaemia. *Lancet* i, 1208–1211.

Treasure, C.B., Klein, J.L., Weintraub, W.S. *et al.* (1995) Beneficial effects of cholesterol lowering therapy on the coronary endothelium in patients with coronary artery disease. *N. Engl. J. Med.* 332, 481–487.

Tunstall-Pedoe, H. (1991) The Dundee coronary risk disk for management of change in risk factors. *Br. Med. J.* 303, 744–7.

Turpeinen, O. (1979) Effect of cholesterol-lowering diet on mortality from coronary heart disease and other causes. *Circulation* 59, 1–7.

Vega, G.L. and Grundy, S.M. (1986) In vivo evidence for reduced binding of low density lipoproteins to receptors as a cause of primary moderate hypercholesterolaemia. *J. Clin. Invest.* 78, 1410–1414.

Waters, D., Higginson, L., Gladstone, P. *et al.* (1994) Effects of monotherapy with an HMG-CoA reductase inhibitor on the progession of coronary atherosclerosis as assessed by serial quantitative arteriography.

The Canadian Coronary Atherosclerosis Intervention Trial. *Circulation* **89**, 959–968.

Watts, G.F., Lewis, B., Brunt, J.N.H. *et al.* (1992) Effects on coronary artery disease of lipid-lowering diet, or diet plus cholestyramine in the St Thomas' Atherosclerosis Regression Study (STARS). *Lancet* **339**, 563–568.

West of Scotland Coronary Prevention Study Group (1992) A coronary primary prevention study of Scottish men age 45–64 years: trial design. *J. Clin. Epidemiol.* **45**, 849–860.

Williams, R.R., Hunt, S.C., Hopkins, P.H. *et al.* (1988) Familial dyslipidaemic hypertension. Evidence from 58 Utah families for a syndrome present in approximately 12 percent of patients with essential hypertertension. *J. Am. Med. Assoc.* **259**, 3579–3586.

Wong, N.D., Wilson, P.W.F. and Kannel, W.B. (1991) Serum cholesterol as a prognostic factor after myocardial infarction: the Framingham Study. *Ann. Intern. Med.* **115**, 687–693.

Wood, D. (1994) Randomized controlled trial evaluating cardiovascular screening and intervention in general practice: principal results of the British Family Heart Study. *Br. Med. J.* **308**, 313–20.

Wysowski, D.K. and Gross, T.P. (1990) Deaths due to accidents and violence in two recent trials of cholesterol-lowering drugs. *Arch. Intern. Med.* **150**, 2169–2172.

Zilversmit, D.B. (1979). Atherogenesis: a postprandial phenomenon. *Circulation.* **60**, 473–85.

Zimetbaum, P., Frishman, W.H., Ooi, W.L. *et al.* (1992) Plasma lipids and lipoproteins and the incidence of cardiovascular disease in the very elderly: the Bronx Aging Study. *Arterioscler. Thromb.* **12**, 416–423.

Further reading

Betteridge, D.J. (ed.) (1995) *Baillière's Clinical Endocrinology and Metabolism*, Vol. 9, No. 5, *Dyslipidaemia*, Baillière Tindall, London.

Betteridge, D.J. (ed.) (1996) *Lipids: Current Perspectives*, Martin Dunitz, London.

Betteridge, .D.J. and Khan, M. (1995) Review of new guidelines for management of dyslipidaemia, in *Clinical Endocrinology and Metabolism, Vol. 9, No. 4: Dyslipidaemia* (ed. D.J. Betteridge), Baillière Tindall, London.

DiClemente, C., Prochastia, J. *et al.* (1991) The process of smoking cessation: an analysis of pre-contemplation, contemplation and preparation stages of change. *J. Consult. Clin. Psychol.* **59**, 295–304.

Fowler, G. (1993) The Indians' Revenge. *Br. J. Gen. Practice.* **43**, 78–81.

Goldstein, F., Stampfer, M.J. *et al.* (1996) Post menopausal estrogen and progestin use and the risk of cardiovascular disease. *N. Engl. J. Med.* **335**, 453–61.

Grady, D. *et al.* (1992) Hormone therapy to prevent disease and prolong life in post menopausal women. *Ann. Intern. Med.* **117**, 1016–37.

Haq, I. *et al.* (1995) Targeting lipid-lowering drug therapy for primary prevention of coronary disease: an updated Sheffield table. *Lancet.* **348**, 387–8.

Kannel, W.B. (1990) Contribution of the Framingham Heart Study to preventive cardiology. *J. Am. Coll. Cardiol.* **15**, 206–211.

Keys, A. (1970) Coronary heart disease in seven countries. *Circulation.* **41** (suppl. 1).

Krentz (1996) Insulin resistance. *Br. Med. J.* **313**, 1385–9.

Lawrence, M., Neil, A., Fowler, G. and Mont, D. (1996) *Prevention of Cardiovascular Disease: an evidence based approach*, Oxford University Press, Oxford.

Lindsay, G.M. and Gaw, A. (eds) (1997) *Coronary Heart Disease Prevention: A Handbook for the Health Care Team*, Churchill Livingstone, London.

Mann, J. *et al.* (1988) British National Lipid Screening Project. *Br. Med. J.* **296**, 1702–6.

Marmot, M. and Elliott, P. (eds) (1992) *Coronary Heart Disease Epidemiology. From Aetiology to Public Health*, Oxford Medical Publications.

Pharoah, P. and Hollingworth, W. (1996) Cost effectiveness of lowering cholesterol concentration with statins in patients with and without pre-existing coronary heart disease: life table method applied to health authority population. *Br. Med. J.* **312**, 1443–8.

Poulter, N., Sever, P. and Thom, S. (eds) (1996) *Cardiovascular Disease: Practical Issues for Prevention*, (2nd edn), Lynne Whitfield, Surbiton.

Scriver, C.R., Beaudet, A.L., Sly, W.S. and Valle, D. (eds) (1995) *The Metabolic and Molecular Bases of Inherited Disease*, 7th edn, McGraw Hill, New York.

Shaper, A.G., Pocock, S.J., Walker, M. *et al.* (1981) British Regional Heart Study. *Br. Med. J.* **283**, 179–186.

Sharp, I. (ed.) (1994) *Coronary Heart Disease: Are Women Special?* National Forum for Coronary Heart Disease Prevention.

Silagy, C. *et al.* (1994) Meta-analysis of efficacy of nicotine replacement therapies in smoking cessation. *Lancet.* **343**, 139–42.

Stamler, J. (1986) Findings of the Multiple Risk Factor Intervention Trial. *J. Am. Med. Assoc.* **254**, 2823–2828.

Syränne, M. and Taskinen, M. (1997) Lipids and Lipoproteins as coronary risk factors in non-insulin dependent diabetes mellitus. *Lancet.* **350** (suppl. 1), 20–3.

Ulbricht, T. and Southgate, D. (1991) Coronary Heart Disease: seven dietary factors. *Lancet.* **338**, 985–92.

Index